SOUTH   T

COOKBOOK

Learn to Make the Most Delicious and Simplified Southern
Recipes

(Loose Weight and Get Healthy the South Beach Way)

Linda Jansen

Published by Alex Howard

South Beach Diet Cookbook: Learn to Make the Most Delicious and Simplified Southern Recipes (Loose Weight and Get Healthy the South Beach Way)

ISBN 978-1-77485-015-2

Legal & Disclaimer

The information contained in this book is not designed to replace or take the place of any form of medicine or professional medical advice. The information in this book has been provided for educational and entertainment purposes only.

Table of contents

Part 1

Introduction

The South Beach Diet is now a home-delivery program broken into two phases. There's no counting calories the bulk of your food shows up at your door. You'll receive three meals a day, plus snacks if you've ordered the "tier 2" program. The diet lasts as long as you want it depends on your weight-loss goal.

Phase one is the weight-loss phase. You will stay in this phase until you reach your desired weight-loss goal or you want more flexibility in your food choices. In phase one, you will limit daily net carbs to 50 grams. You'll include high-quality protein (such as fish, shellfish, chicken, turkey, lean beef and soy) and nonstarchy vegetables. You may include very small quantities of beans and legumes, and extremely small amounts of high-fiber fruits like berries and high-protein whole grains like quinoa.

You will jumpstart phase one with a "Body Reboot," lasting one week and including three meals and three snacks each day. On most day, you will include South Beach Diet prepared breakfasts, lunches, dinners and two snacks (a bar and a shake.) Twice each week, you will include two DIY meals, which can be cooked at home or eaten out. In addition to South Beach Diet prepared foods, you'll need to purchase some of your own fresh grocery foods to complete the plan. After the Body Reboot week, you will continue on to phase one. Lower-carb alcohol, such as a glass of dry red wine, is OK, but it should be limited to no more than two servings a week.

Phase two, the maintenance phase, is your lifelong healthy way to eat. You'll begin to reintroduce more "good carbs," such as whole grains, low-sugar fruits and starchy vegetables. You'll also begin to increase your daily net carbs with a goal between 75 and 100 grams per day. You'll keep up a high protein intake, representing at least 25% of your daily calories, to maintain muscle mass. Although no food is off-limits, some individuals such as people who are insulin-resistant or postmenopausal women may have more success by continuing to limit their carbs. During this phase, you can continue ordering South Beach products a la carte, and you're encouraged to use portion-control containers and the program guide to transition to this stage.

South Beach is launching a keto-friendly diet approach planned for late 2019. The South Beach Keto Diet Friendly plan includes elements of the ketogenic diet low carbs and high fat but does not require you to be as strict in limiting your carbohydrate intake, allowing for more variety in the diet. The South Beach Diet Keto Friendly approach does not require you to be or stay in ketosis to see the weight-loss benefits.

The South Beach Diet, which is named after a glamorous area of Miami, is sometimes called a modified low-carbohydrate diet. The South Beach Diet is lower in carbs (carbohydrates) and higher in protein and healthy fats than is a typical eating plan. But it's not a strict low-carb diet.

There is also a keto (ketogenic) version of the South Beach diet. Ketogenic diets include very few carbs. The goal of a ketogenic diet is to force the body to use fat for energy instead of carbohydrates or protein.

The South Beach Diet

The South Beach Diet was created in the mid-1990s by Dr. Arthur Agatston, a Florida-based cardiologist. His work in heart disease research led to the development of the Agatston score, which measures the amount of calcium in the coronary arteries.

According to published interviews, Dr. Agatston observed that patients on the Atkins Diet were losing weight and belly fat, while those on low-fat, high-carb diets were struggling to achieve results.

However, he was uncomfortable with the high amount of saturated fat allowed on the Atkins Diet, especially for people with heart disease. In addition, he didn't believe in restricting high-fiber foods with "good carbs," like fruit and whole grains.

Dr. Agatston wanted to create a diet that allowed overweight, diabetic and prediabetic individuals to easily lose weight and reduce their risk of heart disease. Therefore, he developed the South Beach Diet, which is rich in low-glycemic-index carbs, lean proteins and unsaturated fats.

After losing weight and belly fat when he tried the diet out on himself, he began prescribing it to his patients, who reported similar results.

SUMMARY:

The South Beach Diet is a lower-carb diet that emphasizes lean meats, unsaturated fats and low-glycemic-index carbs. It was created by cardiologist Dr. Arthur Agatston.

How Does the South Beach Diet Work

The South Beach Diet has three different phases: two for weight loss and a third for weight maintenance.

Purpose

The purpose of the South Beach Diet is to change the overall balance of the foods you eat to encourage weight loss and a healthy lifestyle. The South Beach Diet says it's a healthy way of eating whether you want to lose weight or not.

Why you might follow the South Beach Diet

You might choose to follow the South Beach Diet because you:

Enjoy the types and amounts of food featured in the diet

Want a diet that restricts certain carbs and fats to help you lose weight

Want to change your overall eating habits

Want a diet you can stick with for life

Like the related South Beach Diet products, such as cookbooks and diet foods

Check with your doctor or dietitian before starting any weight-loss diet, especially if you have any health concerns.

Diet details

The South Beach Diet says that its balance of complex carbs, lean protein and healthy fats makes it a nutrient-dense, fiber-rich diet that you can follow for a lifetime of healthy eating. Food sources of complex carbs, or so-called good carbs, include fruit, vegetables, whole grains, beans and legumes. Simple carbs, or "bad" carbs, include sugar, syrup and baked goods made from refined white flour.

The South Beach Diet also teaches you about the different kinds of dietary fats and encourages you to limit unhealthy fats while eating more foods with healthier monounsaturated fats. The South Beach Diet emphasizes the benefits of fiber and whole grains and encourages you to include fruits and vegetables in your eating plan.

Carbohydrates

The South Beach Diet is lower in carbohydrates than is a typical eating plan, but not as low as a strict low-carb diet. On a typical eating plan, about 45% to 65% of your daily calories come from carbohydrates. Based on a 2,000-calorie-a-day diet, this amounts to about 225 to 325 grams of carbohydrates a day.

In the final maintenance phase of the South Beach Diet, you can get as much as 28% of your daily calories from carbohydrates, or about 140 grams of carbohydrates a day. A strict low-carb diet might restrict your carb intake to as little as 20 to 100 grams a day. The keto version of the South Beach diet limits carbs to 40 grams a day during phase 1, and 50 grams during phase 2.

Exercise

The South Beach Diet has evolved over time and now recommends exercise as an important part of your lifestyle. The South Beach Diet says that regular exercise will boost your metabolism and help prevent weight-loss plateaus.

Phases of the South Beach Diet

The South Beach Diet has three phases:

Phase 1. This two-week phase is designed to eliminate cravings for foods high in sugar and refined starches to jump-start weight loss. You cut out almost all carbohydrates from your diet, including pasta, rice, bread and fruit. You can't drink fruit juice or any alcohol. You focus on eating lean protein, such as seafood, skinless poultry, lean beef and soy products. You can also eat high-fiber vegetables, low-fat dairy and foods with healthy, unsaturated fats, including avocados, nuts and seeds.

Phase 2. This is a long-term weight-loss phase. You begin adding back some of the foods that were prohibited in phase 1, such as whole-grain breads, whole-wheat pasta, brown rice, fruits and more vegetables. You stay in this phase until you reach your goal weight.

Phase 3. This is a maintenance phase meant to be a healthy way to eat for life. You continue to follow the lifestyle principles you learned in the two previous phases. You can eat all types of foods in moderation.

A typical day's menu on the South Beach Diet
Here's a look at what you might eat during a typical day in phase 1 of the South Beach Diet:

Breakfast. Breakfast might be an omelet with smoked salmon or baked eggs with spinach and ham, along with a cup of coffee or tea.

Lunch. Lunch might be a vegetable salad with scallops or shrimp, along with iced tea or sparkling water.

Dinner. Dinner may feature grilled tuna or pork paired with grilled vegetables and a salad.

Dessert. The diet encourages you to enjoy a dessert, such as a ricotta cheesecake or chilled espresso custard, even in phase 1.

Snacks. You can enjoy snacks during the day, too, such as a Muenster cheese and turkey roll-up or roasted chickpeas.

Phase 1

Phase 1 lasts 14 days.

It's considered the strictest phase because it limits fruit, grains and other higher-carb foods in order to decrease blood sugar and insulin levels, stabilize hunger and reduce cravings. Most people can expect to lose 8–13 pounds (3.5–6 kg) of body weight during this phase.

During phase 1, you consume three meals per day composed of lean protein, non-starchy vegetables and small amounts of healthy fat and legumes. In addition, you consume two mandatory snacks per day, preferably a combination of lean protein and vegetables.

Phase 2

This phase begins on day 15 and should be maintained for as many weeks as necessary to achieve your goal weight. You can expect to lose 1–2 pounds (0.5–1 kg) per week during this phase, on average. During phase 2, all foods from phase 1 are allowed, plus limited portions of fruit and "good carbs," such as whole grains and certain types of alcohol.

Phase 3

Once you achieve your target weight, you advance to phase three. In this stage, although the phase-2 guidelines should be the basis for your lifestyle, occasional treats are allowed and no foods are truly off limits.

However, if you overindulge and start putting on weight, Dr. Agatston recommends returning to phase 1 for one to two weeks before returning to phase three. In The South Beach Diet Supercharged, Dr. Agatston also recommends regular exercise and provides a three-phase fitness program to accompany the diet phases.

SUMMARY:

The South Beach Diet consists of three phases: a low-carb phase for rapid weight loss, a less restrictive phase for more gradual weight loss and a third phase for weight maintenance.

Phase 1: Foods to Include

Please note that the guidelines for all phases are from the book, The South Beach Diet Supercharged. The guidelines on the South Beach Diet website may be different.

Lean Protein

Although portions aren't limited, the diet recommends slowly consuming a small portion and returning for seconds if you are still hungry.

Lean beef, pork, lamb, veal and game
Skinless chicken and turkey breast
Fish and shellfish
Turkey bacon and pepperoni
Eggs and egg whites
Soy-based meat substitutes
Low-fat hard cheese, ricotta cheese and cottage cheese
Buttermilk, low-fat milk, plain or Greek yogurt, kefir and soy milk, limited to 2 cups (473 ml) daily
Non-Starchy Vegetables
Consume a minimum of 4 1/2 cups daily.

All vegetables are allowed except beets, carrots, corn, turnips, yams, peas, white potatoes and most types of winter squash.

Legumes

Limit these to 1/3–1/2 cup per day, cooked, unless otherwise noted.

Black beans, kidney beans, pinto beans, navy beans, garbanzo beans and other bean varieties

Split peas and black-eyed peas

Lentils

Edamame and soybeans

Hummus, limited to 1/4 cup

Nuts and Seeds

Limit these to 1 oz (28 grams) per day.

Almonds, cashews, macadamias, pecans, pistachios, walnuts and other nuts

Nut butters, limited to 2 tbsp

Flaxseeds, chia seeds, sesame seeds, pumpkin seeds and other seeds

Oils and Fats

Limited to 2 tbsp of oil per day. Monounsaturated oils are encouraged.

Monounsaturated oils, such as olive, canola, macadamia and avocado oils

Vegetable and seed oils, such as corn, flaxseed, grapeseed, peanut, safflower, sesame and soybean oil

Alternative Fat Choices

Each serving is equivalent to 2 tbsp of healthy oils.

Avocado, limited to 2/3 of one fruit

Trans-fat-free margarine, limited to 2 tbsp

Low-fat mayonnaise, limited to 2 tbsp

Regular mayonnaise, limited to 1 tbsp

Salad dressing with less than 3 grams sugar, limited to 2 tbsp

Olives, limited to 20–30, depending on size

Sweet Treats

Limit consumption to 100 calories or fewer per day.

Sugar-free or unsweetened cocoa or chocolate syrup

Sugar-free gelatin, jams and jellies

Sugar-free candies, popsicles or gum

Sugar substitutes, including Stevia, artificial sweeteners and sugar alcohols like xylitol and erythritol

Condiments

You may eat unlimited quantities of these foods, unless otherwise noted.

Broth

Herbs, spices, horseradish, mustard, lemon juice or salsa

All vinegars, with balsamic limited to 1 tbsp

Light coconut milk, limited 1/4 cup (59 ml)

Soy sauce, steak sauce or miso, limited to 1 1/2 tsp (7 ml)

Cream, whole milk or half and half, limited to 1 tbsp

Light sour cream or cream cheese, limited to 2 tbsp
Light whipped topping, limited to 2 tbsp

Beverages

You may drink unlimited quantities of these beverages, although drinking your caffeine in moderation is advised.

Coffee, regular or decaffeinated
Tea, regular, decaffeinated or herbal
Sugar-free sodas
Sugar-free drink mixes
Tomato juice or vegetable juice

Phase 1: Foods to Avoid

Certain fatty foods and those high in carbs, including fruits and grains, are not allowed in phase 1. These include:

Fatty meat and poultry
Butter and coconut oil
Whole milk
Foods made with refined sugar
Honey, maple syrup and agave nectar
Grains
All fruits and fruit juice
Beets, carrots, corn, turnips, yams, peas, white potatoes and winter squash
Alcohol

Phases 2 and 3: Foods to Include

Phase 2 includes all phase 1 foods and gradually adds in higher-carb foods, beginning with one daily serving of fruit and whole grains or starchy vegetables for the first week.

On the 14th day of phase 2 and thereafter, you may consume up to three servings of fruit and four servings of whole grains and starchy vegetables per day.

An occasional alcoholic drink is also allowed, although choices are limited to light beer and dry wine.

Once you've achieved your goal weight, you move to phase three for maintenance. During this phase, you should generally follow the guidelines from phase 2.

However, you can include "treat" foods occasionally, since no foods are completely off limits.

Fruits

Consume 1–3 servings per day. All fresh and frozen fruits are allowed except dates, figs, pineapple, raisins and watermelon.
A serving size is one small piece of fruit, half a grapefruit or 3/4 cup (about 115 grams) berries, cherries or grapes.

Whole Grains and Starchy Vegetables

Consume 1–4 servings per day.

Except where noted, one serving size is 1/2 cup cooked starchy vegetables, 1 slice bread or 1/2 cup cooked grains.

Peas

Rutabaga

Sweet potatoes and yams

Turnips

Winter squash, limited to 3/4 cup

Whole-grain hot cereal

Whole-grain cold cereal, limited to 1 cup

Whole-grain bread

Brown or wild rice

Whole-grain pasta, quinoa, couscous or farro

Taro, limited to 1/3 cup

Popcorn, limited to 3 cups

Whole-grain bagel, limited to 1/2 small

Pita bread, limited to 1/2 pita

Corn or whole-grain tortilla, limited to 1 small

Alcohol

One daily serving of dry wine or an occasional light beer is allowed.

Light beer, limited to 12 oz (355 ml)

Wine, dry red or white, limited to 4 oz (118 ml)

Phases 2 and 3: Foods to Avoid

Phase 2 of the South Beach Diet discourages intake of fatty meats, saturated fat and foods high in refined or natural sugar. Try to avoid:

Fatty meat and poultry
Butter and coconut oil
Whole milk
Foods made with refined flour or sugar
Honey, maple syrup, agave nectar
Fruit juice
Beets, corn and white potatoes
Dates, figs, pineapple, raisins and watermelon
Alcohol other than light beer and dry wine

Sample Days on the Diet

Here are sample meal plans for phase 1 and phase 2 of the South Beach Diet, to give you a snapshot of what a typical day might look like.

Phase 1 Sample Day

Breakfast: 3 eggs and 1 cup kale cooked with 1 tsp olive oil

Snack: 1 oz (28 grams) string cheese with bell pepper slices

Lunch: Roasted salmon and asparagus salad with mustard vinaigrette

Snack: Celery sticks with 2 tsp peanut butter

Dinner: Lean steak with broccoli

Phase 2 Sample Day
Breakfast: Quick and easy peanut butter oatmeal
Snack: 1 cup cucumber slices with 1/4 cup hummus
Lunch: Apple-walnut chicken salad
Snack: Cottage cheese with cherry tomatoes
Dinner: Pork fajitas with 1/3 cup guacamole

There are hundreds of recipes available for all three phases of the South Beach Diet, including many with ingredients that are cheap, tasty and easy to find.

SUMMARY:

You can find many recipes for the South Beach Diet, with the sample days above indicating how the days might look.

Benefits of the South Beach Diet

There are several benefits of the South Beach diet, including its ability to produce weight loss without hunger. Research, including an analysis of 24 studies, has consistently shown that high-protein, low-carb diets are effective for weight loss.

Part of this is due to protein's ability to increase your metabolic rate. In addition, protein helps modify hormone levels that reduce hunger and promote fullness, so you end up naturally eating less.

What's more, gradually adding small amounts of healthy carbs back into your diet may promote continued weight loss in some people and make it easier for them to stick to the diet long-term.

In one study, overweight and obese people with metabolic syndrome followed the South Beach Diet for 12 weeks.

By the end of the study, they had lost 11 pounds (5.2 kg) and 2 inches (5.1 cm) from around their waists, on average. They also experienced significant decreases in fasting insulin and an increase in the fullness hormone CCK.

The South Beach Diet encourages a high intake of fatty fish like salmon and other foods that fight inflammation, such as leafy greens and cruciferous veggies.

In addition, it recommends dieters regularly consume eggs, nuts, seeds, extra virgin olive oil and other foods that have been shown to protect heart health.

The book makes meal planning easy and pleasurable by providing two weeks of sample menus and recipes for each phase. There are also hundreds of recipes available online for phase 1 and phase 2 meals.

SUMMARY:

The South Beach Diet may help you lose weight and belly fat, reduce insulin levels, increase hormone levels that promote fullness and help protect heart health.

Downsides of the South Beach Diet

Unfortunately, the South Beach Diet also has a couple of drawbacks. The main issue is that it may be overly restrictive with respect to the amounts and types of fats allowed.

In addition, it allows potentially harmful types of fat, such as soybean oil and safflower oil, which are extremely high in omega-6 fatty acids.

Although it's important to get some omega-6 fats in your diet, if you're like most people, you probably already get far more than you need.

In contrast, if you eat a Western Diet, it's likely you get too little of the anti-inflammatory omega-3 fats found in fatty fish like salmon, sardines and mackerel.

Consuming a high ratio of omega-6 to omega-3 fats has been linked to inflammation, heart disease and other health problems. In contrast, butter and coconut oil aren't included on the South Beach Diet because they are high in saturated fat.

However, coconut oil has been credited with several health benefits, including weight loss, a reduction in belly fat and better heart health markers in overweight and obese adults.

In addition, most comprehensive reviews of studies have found no association between saturated fat intake and an increased risk of heart disease.

On the other hand, other large reviews have found that replacing a portion of saturated fat with unsaturated fat could potentially reduce the risk of heart disease (18Trusted Source, 19Trusted Source).

Overall, choosing less processed fat and eating plenty of fish high in omega-3 fats may be more important for heart health than restricting saturated fat.

SUMMARY:

The South Beach Diet may be overly restrictive by prohibiting many saturated fat sources and limiting fat intake overall. In addition, it allows the use of processed vegetable oils.

Is the South Beach Diet Safe and Sustainable

The South Beach Diet is a healthy way of eating that is far lower in carbs than conventional low-fat diets. It also encourages dieters to eat mainly unprocessed foods, liberal amounts of vegetables and healthy, high-fiber carb sources.

However, the diet allows processed vegetable oils, which could pose health risks. Nevertheless, you can avoid this drawback by choosing unprocessed monounsaturated fats like extra virgin olive oil, avocado oil or macadamia oil instead. All this being said, the South Beach Diet is likely a sustainable way of eating. Many people have reported losing weight and keeping it off by following the diet.

Yet in the end, the most effective diet for weight loss is whichever one you can easily stick with long-term.

The Possible Pros of Following the South Beach Diet "This plan is presented very simply, no measuring for many of the foods is necessary, especially at the beginning," "Due to the strictness of phase 1, some people could have a significant amount of weight loss in the first two weeks, [such as] 8 to 12 pounds. Phase 1 could help stop cravings for highly refined carbs, and the foods recommended throughout the plan are heart healthy." Blood sugar control has the added bonus of helping control type 2 diabetes if you already have it.

The Possible Cons of Following the South Beach Diet
The South Beach Diet might represent the ultimate eating plan for some, but it may not be perfect for everyone. For one thing, Schmidt says the diet doesn't provide enough calcium, which is especially important for women because they are more prone to osteoporosis, or bone loss. Getting a sufficient amount of calcium in your diet can help build and maintain strong bones and ward off the bone disease.

More on Building Strong Bones

Although guidelines include 2 cups of dairy (like milk and cheese) per day, this isn't enough. "You absolutely need a calcium supplement, 500 milligrams with vitamin D, in the morning and in the evening. I also don't like the idea that there's no fruit and no starch during phase 1," though this is less of a problem if you're only on it for the two weeks.

Phase 1 is stringent and, because of the limited nature of certain foods, some people might have a tough time following it, especially when they're away from home. "There are no specific recommendations for portions for many of the food groups." This could lead to overeating or even undereating.

And some studies haven't found any benefit of the South Beach Diet over other popular diet programs: For example, a review published in November 2014 in Circulation: Cardiovascular Quality and Outcomes looked at the effectiveness of the Atkins diet, the South Beach diet, the Zone diet, and the Weight Watchers diet, and researchers did not find evidence that any one plan was significantly more effective than the others. (Of them all, at 12 months, the Weight Watchers diet appeared most effective at reducing weight.)

What to Expect on the South Beach Diet

The South Beach Diet touts many benefits, including substantial weight loss, stabilized blood sugar, reduced cravings, and increased energy. When following the South Beach Diet, you can expect a drastic change to your diet, at least in the first phase.

There are three phases of the South Beach Diet. Phase 1 is the most restrictive (no fruit, grains, starches, or alcohol) and lasts one to two weeks to help your body reboot and get used to burning fat instead of carbs for fuel. After that, you'll be able to slowly add foods with carbohydrates back into your diet.

It's important to note that the South Beach Diet includes three phases, and the foods you can and cannot eat differ as you move through the phases. Here's a rundown of what you can and can't eat during phases one, two and three.

Phase 1

During Phase 1 of the South Beach Diet, you will be able to eat many of the foods you currently enjoy, including ground beef and a variety of vegetables. These foods are low on the glycemic index and are supposed to help you to eliminate cravings for starchy carbohydrates and sweets.

You'll cut carbohydrates during this phase, and that will help you to reduce excess water weight. You may see a five-pound change on the scale or even more in the span of a week.

Compliant Foods (Phase 1)

During Phase 1, these are the foods and ingredients you can incorporate into your diet:

Meats and poultry: You can enjoy a range of protein sources on the South Beach Diet, as long as you focus on meats low in fat, especially saturated fats. Enjoy boiled ham, lean cuts of beef, such as flank steak or eye of round, skinless turkey and chicken breast, Canadian and turkey bacon, pork tenderloin, lower-fat and lower-sodium lunch meats including lean deli roast beef or smoked turkey.

Seafood: You can eat all types of fish seafood on the South Beach Diet, but try to limit your intake of high-mercury fish and seafood.

Eggs: The South Beach Diet permits whole eggs and egg whites, so you can still enjoy your morning omelet.

Soy products: If you're vegetarian or vegan, you can opt for soy-based meat substitutes such as soy bacon or soy crumbles.

Beans: Beans are a great source of fiber and plant-based protein, and you can eat many varieties on the South Beach Diet, including black-eyed peas, great northern beans, chickpeas, and pinto beans.

Nuts: Snack on nuts such as almonds, cashews, and macadamia nuts, but you must limit your intake to one serving per day.

Non-starchy vegetables: Any non-starchy vegetable is a go on the South Beach Diet. Incorporate a lot of leafy greens, sprouts, lettuce, okra, peppers, and cruciferous veggies like broccoli.

Dairy: You're encouraged to enjoy full-fat dairy rather than low- or no-fat, because many manufacturers add sugar to make up for the lost flavor in low-fat options.

Healthy fats: Each day, you can consume up to 2 tablespoons of healthy oils like olive oil; avocado (1/3 avocado equals one tablespoon of your healthy oil intake); and 2 tablespoons of salad dressing with less than 3 grams of sugar.

Non-compliant Foods (Phase 1)
Here's what you'll want to avoid:

Fatty cuts of meat: You should avoid fatty meats like brisket and prime rib, dark meat from poultry, poultry with skin, duck meat, and chicken wings and legs. You should also avoid sugary meats such as honey-baked ham and beef jerky.

Starchy vegetables: During Phase 1 of the South Beach Diet, you should avoid starchy vegetables such as potatoes and sweet potatoes, corn, beets, yams, turnips, and green peas.

Grains and starches: You can't eat any carbohydrates from grain sources during Phase 1. This includes bread, crackers, chips, pretzels, oatmeal, cereal, pasta, granola, rice, bagels, buns, and other sources.

Alcohol: Alcohol—including beer, hard liquor, wine, and mixed drinks—is off-limits during phase one.

Sugar-sweetened beverages: Sports drinks, energy drinks, sodas, juices, and other beverages that contain sugar aren't allowed on the South Beach Diet. Ideally, you should also avoid artificially sweetened beverages as they can contribute to bloating and digestive discomfort.

Desserts: Refrain from eating cookies, cakes, ice cream, candy, frozen yogurt, and other sugary desserts during Phase 1 of the South Beach Diet.

Phase 2

In the first two weeks on South Beach, you eat from a list of foods, and that's it. After the first phase, it's time to start individualizing the diet for your own body and tastes.

The goal of Phase 2 of the South Beach Diet is to find the right carb level for you. This is done by gradually reintroducing some high nutrient, high fiber, low glycemic carbohydrates into your diet. How much and what types will vary between individuals. During this phase, weight loss will likely slow to one to two pounds per week, so keep this in mind as well. Phase 2 of the South Beach Diet lasts until you reach your goal weight.

Week One

The plan of the first week of Phase 2 is to add one serving of a carbohydrate food to each day, experimenting to see how you feel. Chances are this first food will not be problematic.

What should the food be? Generally, it is a serving from the approved fruit list or a serving of a low-glycemic starch. Dr. Arthur Agatson, the creator of the South Beach Diet, recommends that if you choose fruit to have it at lunch or dinner. He thinks that fruit at breakfast is more likely to induce cravings.

If you choose an approved whole grain, he recommends a high fiber, low-carb cereal such as Fiber One, All Bran with extra fiber, or slow-cooked oatmeal (not instant). If you are having cereal for breakfast, be sure to include some protein as well.

Week Two

In the second week, you will add a second daily serving of carbohydrate food, as above. That means you will be eating one serving of fruit and one serving of a high-fiber starchy food each day this week, in addition to all the other foods.

Week Three

During the third week, you will again add a serving of carbohydrate food daily if you can tolerate it without weight gain or cravings. It's also probably a good idea to talk a bit about bread at this point. Look for bread with at least 3 grams of fiber per serving—bread made specifically to be low-carb usually has more fiber and less starch. If bread is a problem for you, at this point or later, choose a grain that is not ground into flour, such as brown rice, and see if you tolerate it better.

Week Four

Add another serving of carbohydrates. At this point, you may be getting near the limit of carbohydrates you can eat and continue to lose weight and some people will have passed that limit. Watch carefully for the signs of carb cravings.

Week Five

If you can handle it, add another serving of carbohydrates. At this point, your menus should look like Phase 1 meals but with the addition of two or three servings each of fruit, starches or grains, and dairy. Lunch and dinner should each have at least 2 cups of vegetables along with a serving of protein.

Week Six

If you are still able to add carbohydrates, you will be eating three servings of fruit and three servings of grains or starches. If this is too much carbohydrate, try substituting more non-starchy vegetables. At this point, you have transitioned completely into Phase 2 of the South Beach Diet. This is the way you should eat until you reach your goal weight and are ready for Phase 3.

Phase 3

This is the lifelong endpoint of the South Beach Diet. You have now attained your goal weight. But even more important for long-term success, you have learned to eat and enjoy healthier food. You can celebrate your success but you need to make the most of what you learned along the way.

What Can You Eat in Phase 3

The short answer is that you can eat anything you want. But that depends on what you want to eat, and how much. You can't forget the lessons you learned in Phase 1 and 2, making better choices to enjoy lean protein, vegetables, healthy oils, and appropriate portions. Desserts, alcohol, sugary drinks, and fatty meats should remain off-limits for the best results.

You will be able to determine the number of carbs you can add back into your diet without gaining weight. If you see your weight increase, cut back on carbs. If you need to lose weight, you can start the Phases over again.

How Long to Follow Phase 3

By the time you reach Phase 3, you will have learned all the skills you need to maintain your goal weight, and you can maintain Phase 3 for good if you wish.

Recommended Timing

The South Beach Diet doesn't enforce any specific timing for your meals or snacks. Rather, people on the diet are simply encouraged to eat up to six times per day: three meals, and three snacks, a pretty typical recommendation.

It's a good idea to space your meals and snacks out by two to four hours going too long without food can lead to hunger pangs, which can lead to overeating. Don't forget to drink plenty of water before, during, and after your meals. Staying hydrated will help you feel fuller for longer.

Set Yourself Up for Success

If you're concerned that you won't be able to survive the first stage of the South Beach Diet, you're not alone. Many people find the list of Phase 1 foods to be too restrictive. But if you want to make the diet work, there are a few ways to set yourself up for success:

Fill your pantry with your favorite Phase 1 diet foods: Get the complete list, find the foods that make you most happy, and fill your kitchen with those items. Schedule an hour (at least) to visit the grocery store and check out areas of the market that you generally skip. You might find new foods and flavors to explore.

Clean out your kitchen: Make sure all foods that are not allowed are thrown away. That means that you clean out your refrigerator and pantry and set up your kitchen for weight loss success. Having the wrong foods in your kitchen will only make the first phase more difficult.

Start the South Beach Diet exercise plan: You'll be less likely to crave the Phase 1 diet foods you can't eat if you fill your day with healthy activity that gets you away from the kitchen. The South Beach exercise program is specifically designed for beginners who want to burn calories and stay active. And if you follow the plan precisely, you won't do too much too soon and get hungry or tired as a result.

Phase 1 Tips

Once you know which foods to eat and which foods to avoid during Phase 1 of the South Beach Diet, use these helpful tips to eat better and lose weight.

Don't rely on "healthy" foods: Just because a food is healthy, doesn't mean that it is good for your diet during Phase 1. In fact, many healthy foods are not allowed during Phase 1 of the South Beach Diet. Fruit is a good example. Whole fruit contains fiber and other healthy vitamins and minerals. But because fruit contains a lot of sugar (fructose) it is not allowed during Phase 1. Homemade baked goods are another food to ditch during Phase 1. Stick to the food list to make meal and snack choices—even when the menu options sound healthy.

Stick to unprocessed foods: The tricky thing about Phase 1 is that you have to avoid certain foods—like sugar but also any product that contains that food as an ingredient. If you eat heavily processed packaged foods, you'll have to scour the ingredients list of every product you buy to uncover hidden ingredients. It's easier and healthier to eat whole foods in their natural state.

Measure portion sizes: Portion size matters on every diet. It is especially important during Phase 1 of The South Beach diet if you want to lose a lot of weight. Many items on the Phase 1 food list have suggested serving sizes. Nuts, for example, are limited to one serving per day and each variety of nut has a different serving size. Only 2 cups of dairy products are allowed each day and sweet treats are limited to 75–100 calories per day.

Get creative in the kitchen. You'll be able to eat more food and you'll be less hungry if you cook your own healthy South Beach Diet foods. There are plenty of recipes online and in the book. Try new recipes and experiment with new flavors. It will help you to keep your mind off of the foods that are not allowed during Phase 1.

Plan meals and snacks in advance. It's going to be natural to want to fall back into your old eating habits during Phase 1 of the South Beach Diet. In social situations and during stressful moments you're going to be tempted to reach for the foods that used to bring you comfort. So how do you combat those cravings? Be prepared. Plan your meals and snacks in advance so that you always have Phase 1 foods on hand.

Phase 2 Tips

You may want to keep a food journal during Phase 2 to set yourself up for success in Phase 3, when you no longer rely solely on food lists. You'll have much more control over what you eat, when, and how often.

If you learn as much as possible during Phase 2 about the foods that make you feel good, the foods that trigger cravings, and the foods you're tempted to overeat, you'll be more likely to continue your healthy South Beach Diet eating habits in a way that is satisfying and sustainable for long-term health.

Phase 3 Tips

You first will have gone through the restrictive food list in Phase 1, which cuts out most of the carbohydrates from your diet. This is a week-long phase to get you out of cravings for high-sugar foods. For many people, that is the bulk of their diet before they start the South Beach Diet, so it can be quite a hurdle to overcome.

But in the two weeks on Phase 1, you also learn to eat (and hopefully enjoy) healthier options. This re-education of your palate and change to your plate will be something you carry into Phase 2 and 3. lean protein, high-fiber vegetables, low-fat dairy products. Here you also learned to use unsaturated fats, nuts, seeds, and avocados.

You probably also re-educated yourself as to what a healthy food portion was, so you will know to look at a plate whether it contains more food than you should eat in one meal.

Modifications

It is very important to pay attention to your own body's reactions to adding the carbs. If a food sets up cravings or weight gain, back off and try something less glycemic. If you feel fuzzy-headed or lower in energy, ditto.

As always, be attentive to your allergies and sensitivities. The South Beach Diet includes a relatively wide range of foods, especially after the first phase, so you should be able to swap foods as needed.

If cost is a factor for you, don't buy into the paid program. You can save money by buying your groceries and prepping food yourself. On the other hand, if convenience is a bigger factor for you than finances, the paid program with pre-portioned and delivered food may be a good option for you.

You shouldn't attempt Phase 1 if you have a history of disordered eating. Severe food restriction can lead to food fear and labeling of foods as "good" or "bad."

Recipes

Creamy Keto Coffee

Whip up a Creamy Keto Coffee latte that's packed with healthy fats, protein and delicious flavor. Fuel your workouts or your workday with this energizing beverage that features MCT oil and collagen peptides. The addition of egg yolks to this creamy latte will keep you satisfied until lunch.

This creamy coffee recipe is easily whipped up in your blender. Get started by combining two medium egg yolks, one tablespoon of unsalted butter or ghee and one tablespoon of MCT oil in your blender. Pulse to combine, then add two cups of hot dark brewed coffee, one scoop of collage peptides, two teaspoons of an erythritol-based confectioners' sweetener and a half-teaspoon of vanilla extract (optional). Blend for about 30 seconds, then pour your whipped coffee into a mug. Garnish with a sprinkle of cinnamon across the top and serve with a reusable metal straw. Not a fan of raw egg yolks? Feel free to replace them with another tablespoon of butter, ghee, MCT or coconut oil. You can also substitute erythritol with another sweetener that you enjoy.

One serving of this Creamy Keto Coffee contains 183 calories and one gram of net carbs per serving. It counts as one Healthy Fat on the South Beach Diet program. If you're on our keto friendly program, you know that Healthy Fats are very important for your weight loss plan.

Coffee is keto friendly-approved! This bitter beverage contains antioxidants that have been shown to a reduce the risk of heart disease and diabetes, says Healthline. Four cups of coffee a day just might also help you lose weight reducing body fat by about four percent.

Ingredients:

2 medium egg yolks
1 Tbsp. unsalted butter or ghee, melted
1 Tbsp. MCT oil or coconut oil
2 cups hot dark brewed coffee
1 scoop collagen peptides
2 tsp. erythritol-based sweetener (confectioners')
1/2 teaspoon vanilla extract (optional)
1/8 teaspoon cinnamon

Directions:

Combine egg yolks, butter and MCT oil in a blender and pulse to combine.

Add coffee, collagen peptides, erythritol sweetener and vanilla (optional).
Blend for about 30 seconds then serve immediately.

Simple Chicken Soup

This Simple Chicken Soup Recipe is every bit as delicious and cozy as it sounds. Featuring the classic chicken soup ingredients of diced onions, celery, hearty chicken and simmering bone broth, it's got all the traditional flavors that you know and love. Whip up a batch of this delicious soup today and let your family in on the warming action. Or, separate the recipe out into individual containers and enjoy savory satisfaction all week long.

Ingredients:

1 Tbsp. avocado oil
1 small onion, chopped
3 celery stalks, diced
2 garlic cloves, minced
2 tsp. onion powder
2 tsp. garlic powder
5 cups chicken bone broth
1 ½ lb. boneless, skinless chicken breasts, cut into 2-inch strips
2 cups diced tomatoes

Sea salt and pepper, to taste

Directions:

Heat the avocado oil in a large saucepan over medium heat.

Add the onion, celery and minced garlic. Cook for about 5 minutes until the vegetables are tender, stirring often.

Stir in the onion powder and garlic powder. Continue cooking for 30 more seconds.

Add broth, increase heat to high and bring to a rapid simmer.

Add chicken and cook until no longer pink, about 3 minutes.

Stir in tomatoes and bring back to a simmer. Season with salt and pepper to taste. Serve hot.

Nut-Crusted Fish with Herbed Tahini Cheese Sauce

This light and healthy Middle Eastern-inspired fish recipe is packed with protein and clean ingredients. Fresh white fish fillets are covered in a crunchy almond and coconut crust and drizzled with a creamy tahini sauce. We serve it up with a side of shirataki rice for a keto friendly summer meal that's simple yet satisfying. One serving of this Nut-Crusted Fish with Herbed Tahini Cheese Sauce contains 433 calories and seven grams of net carbs.

To spice things up, feel free to substitute the mustard in the sauce with wasabi. You could also add a Vegetable serving to this dish by serving it up with some steamed spinach, Swiss chard or kale. Dark leafy greens are South Beach Diet-approved non-starchy veggies that are great for adding to smoothies, salads and savory dinners. Riced cauliflower is a great swap if you can't find shirataki rice.

Ingredients:

Fish

1/2 cup hazelnuts or almonds, lightly toasted and chopped

1/4 cup unsweetened shredded coconut, lightly toasted

1 tsp. lemon zest

1 tsp. ground sumac, za'atar or dried oregano (optional)

1 1/2 Tbsp. Dijon mustard

1 lemon, juiced

2 Tbsp. olive oil

4 (4.5-oz.) cod, haddock or another firm-fleshed white fish fillets

1 package (7-oz.) shirataki rice, prepared according to package instructions

Tahini Cheese Sauce

1/2 cup tahini

1/4 cup grated parmesan cheese

2 cloves garlic

1 lemon, juiced

1/3 cup mixed fresh herbs (such as flat leaf parsley, dill and cilantro), finely chopped

1/4 cup water (more as needed)

1/2 tsp. harissa (optional)

Directions:

Fish

Preheat the oven to 400F. Lightly grease a rimmed baking sheet. Set aside.

Combine hazelnuts, coconut, lemon zest and sumac (optional) in a small bowl. Set aside.

Pat cod fillets dry then season with salt and pepper to taste.

Stir together Dijon mustard, lemon juice and olive oil in a small bowl, then brush over the cod.

Roll each fillet into the hazelnut mixture and place on the prepared baking sheet.

Bake for 10 to 12 minutes, until the fish is fork tender.

Tahini Cheese Sauce

In a medium mixing bowl, whisk tahini with parmesan cheese, garlic, lemon juice, herbs, and salt and pepper to taste.

Slowly add enough cold water until you get a sauce consistency. Add harissa (optional) and stir to combine.

Drizzle tahini sauce over nut-crusted fish and serve with shirataki rice.

2-Step Chia Yogurt

If you're like us, then you're usually rushing to get out the door on time each morning. This chia pudding recipe with yogurt makes eating healthy feasible with just two simple steps and a few simple ingredients.

This creamy recipe combines the flavors and heartiness of Greek yogurt, chia seeds, almond extract, turmeric and ground cinnamon for a sweet and filling start to your day.

Ingredients:

½ cup or 5.3 oz. Greek yogurt, plain, whole milk
½ Tbsp. chia seeds
1 Tbsp. almonds, unsalted, sliced
¼ tsp. almond extract
½ tsp. turmeric spice
1 pinch ground cinnamon

Directions:

Place all ingredients into container of choice, stirring well to combine.
Enjoy immediately or store in the refrigerator overnight, if you would prefer to allow the chia seeds to absorb the yogurt and expand overnight. Note: the longer you let the yogurt sit, the brighter yellow the yogurt will become.

Spanish Braised Chicken in Creamy Almond Sauce

When you start a low carb diet, keto chicken recipes quickly become a staple on your menu. If you've finally grown tired of eating the same old chicken and veggie dish every night, it's time to spice up your life with our Spanish Braised Chicken in Creamy Almond Sauce! This aromatic one-pot chicken recipe is guaranteed to satisfy your comfort food cravings and add some variety to your week.

The best part about this nutritious and delicious meal is that it's perfect for your weekly meal prep. It tastes just as good the next day, so you can easily make it ahead and re-heat. Keep any leftovers in an airtight container in the refrigerator for up to three days. It's also a freezer friendly dish and can be frozen for up to one month.

One serving of this Spanish Braised Chicken in Creamy Almond Sauce contains 334 calories and seven grams of net carbs.

Ingredients:

2 Tbsp. olive oil
1 lb. boneless skinless chicken thighs
2 Tbsp. unsalted butter

1 medium onion, chopped

3 cloves garlic, minced

2 Tbsp. sundried tomatoes, chopped

1 tsp. smoked paprika

1/2 yellow bell pepper, deseeded and diced

1 serrano or jalapeno pepper, deseeded and diced

1/2 red bell pepper, deseeded and diced

2 sprigs fresh thyme

1 cup chicken broth or water

1/3 cup almonds, chopped

1/4 cup pitted Spanish manzanilla olives (or other green olives), sliced

4 Tbsp. flat leaf parsley, chopped and divided

1 lemon, juiced and zested

Directions:

Heat olive oil in a large skillet over medium-high heat.

Pat chicken thighs dry then season with salt and pepper to taste. Add to pan and cook 4 to 6 minutes per side, until cooked through. Transfer to a plate and set aside.

Add onions to the skillet and cook over medium heat for 3 to 5 minutes, or until translucent.

Stir in garlic, sundried tomatoes, paprika, peppers and thyme. Cook, stirring occasionally, for 4 to 5 minutes until the vegetables are tender.

Add chicken thighs and broth to the skillet and bring to a boil. Reduce the heat to medium-low and cook 12 to 15 minutes, stirring occasionally.

Add almonds, olives, 3 Tablespoons of parsley, lemon zest and lemon juice. Reduce heat to low and simmer for 6 to 8 minutes longer.

Garnish with remaining parsley before serving.

1-Minute Chocolate Ricotta Mousse

Attention all chocolate lovers—This Chocolate Ricotta Mousse recipe is a delightful and healthy snack that is quick and easy to make. Combine the flavorful ingredients in a blender and in a few short minutes, you will be enjoying spoonfuls of chocolatey satisfaction that packs in more than 15 grams of protein!

This healthy take on chocolate mousse will have your taste buds screaming, and your sweet tooth satisfied. With five simple ingredients, this sweet and savory snack can be ready in actual seconds—yes, you heard us correctly, SECONDS! You won't regret blending up this little treat as an evening snack. In fact, don't be surprised if the family is trying to snatch this delicious dessert right out of your hands. This protein-packed piece of chocolate ricotta perfection is sure to become a household regular for you and the family!

Ingredients:

½ cup part-skim ricotta cheese
1 Tbsp. unsweetened vanilla almond milk
1 Tbsp. unsweetened cocoa powder
2-3 drops stevia
1 tsp. cacao nibs

Directions:

In a small blender or food processor whip together ricotta cheese, almond milk, cocoa powder and stevia until smooth. Top with cacao nibs and serve.

No-Bake Strawberry Cheesecake Bliss Balls

Planning your stay-at-home Easter menu? These No-Bake Strawberry Cheesecake Bliss Balls are the perfect addition to your holiday dessert lineup! Add them to your keto friendly Easter basket for a sweet treat that satisfies. You can even shape them like mini Easter eggs to create a seasonal strawberry snack!

These dairy-free, vegan bliss balls taste just like little bites of cheesecake. A small handful of freeze-dried strawberries add tons of fresh berry flavor without adding excess carbs. They hold their shape well at room temperature, so they're great for taking with you for a snack on the go. Try doubling or tripling the recipe and storing in the freezer so you have keto friendly snacks on hand at all times. Simply let sit at room temperature for five minutes to allow them to defrost slightly before eating.

The best part about these mini strawberry cheesecake bites is that they're extremely easy to make! Grab your food processor and combine one cup of raw cashews, two tablespoons of coconut oil, one teaspoon of vanilla extract, two tablespoons of a granulated erythritol-based sweetener and an eighth of a teaspoon of salt. If you are unable to tolerate erythritol, free to swap in another keto friendly sweetener of your choice like stevia or monk fruit. Pulse the food processor until a dough forms, then add a quarter-cup of freeze-dried strawberries. Continue pulsing until the mixture is just combined. Divide the dough into eight equal pieces, then roll them in your hands until you form round or egg-shaped balls. Store them in the refrigerator for up to one week.strawberry cheesecake keto balls

Try swapping in freeze-dried blueberries or raspberries for a fun variation! You can also get creative with other additions, like unsweetened coconut flakes, chia seeds, cacao powder and more. Just make sure to keep track of these additions in your daily food journal. Take a look at our keto friendly Grocery Guide if you need some guidance on Healthy Fats, Proteins, Extras and Free Foods.

This recipe makes eight Strawberry Cheesecake Bliss Balls. One ball contains 129 calories and two grams of net carbs. It counts as one Healthy Fat on your South Beach Diet program. Healthy Fats are essential to a keto friendly diet. However, it's possible to eat too many and go over your daily calories.

Ingredients:

1 cup raw cashews
2 Tbsp. coconut oil
1 tsp. vanilla extract
2 Tbsp. erythritol-based sweetener (granulated)
1/8 tsp. salt
1/4 cup freeze-dried strawberries

Directions:

Pulse cashews, coconut oil, vanilla extract, erythritol and salt in a food processor until a dough forms.
Add berries and pulse again until just combined.
Divide dough into 8 pieces, then roll between the palms of your hands to form balls.
Store in the refrigerator for up to 1 week.

Instant Pot Keto Tuscan Soup

Getting tired of eating the same old Instant Pot recipes over and over again? Add an Italian-inspired meal to your dinner lineup that's filled with robust flavors and clean ingredients. Best of all, this Instant Pot Keto Tuscan Soup recipe is ready to enjoy in just 20 minutes.

Whip up this light yet hearty soup that's packed with comforting ingredients like tender chicken sausage, crispy kale and sautéed garlic and onions. We simmer it all in a creamy, dreamy chicken broth and top it off with grated parmesan cheese and fresh parsley. Your family is sure to love this delicious dinner that provides the classic Italian flavors they love.

Grab your Instant Pot and set it to sauté mode. Add one pound of hot or mild chicken sausage with the casings removed. Cook the sausage until it's lightly browned, about five minutes. Be sure to break it up with a spoon while it's cooking. Next, add in three cloves of minced garlic, one large chopped onion and one teaspoon of dried oregano. Stir constantly for about three minutes until the onions become translucent. Pour in six cups of chicken broth and a half-cup of sun-dried tomatoes. Season with pepper and stir to combine.

Now that the main components of your Tuscan soup are in the Instant Pot, set it to Manual High Pressure for five minutes. When it's finished cooking, do a quick-release. Once it's finished releasing the steam, set your

Instant Pot to sauté mode and add in one bunch of chopped kale (stems removed). Stir the soup for about two minutes until the kale has wilted. Add in three-quarters of a cup of heavy cream and continue cooking for another minute until it's heated through. Season your soup with salt and pepper to taste and remove it from the heat. Garnish with fresh chopped parsley and a quarter-cup of grated parmesan cheese before serving.

Want to make this meal vegetarian? Simply swap in a vegetable broth and use a plant-based Italian sausage instead of chicken. You can also pump up the protein and fiber by adding in some white kidney beans. Just make sure to count this addition towards your daily net carbs for the day.

Ingredients:

1 lb. Italian chicken sausage (hot or mild), casings removed
1 large onion, chopped
3 cloves garlic, minced
1 tsp. dried oregano
½ cup sun-dried tomatoes, drained
Salt and black pepper, to taste
6 cups chicken broth, low sodium
1 bunch kale, leaves stripped from stems and chopped
¾ cup heavy cream
¼ cup grated parmesan

Fresh parsley, chopped (optional)

Directions:

Set a 6-quart Instant Pot to sauté mode. Add the chicken sausage (casings removed) and break it up with a spoon while cooking. Continue cooking until the sausage is lightly browned, about 3-5 minutes.

Add in the garlic, onion and oregano. Stir constantly until the onions become translucent, about 2-3 minutes.

Add in the chicken broth and sun-dried tomatoes. Stir to combine. Season with pepper.

Set the Instant to Pot to Manual High Pressure for 5 minutes. When finished cooking, do a quick-release.

Select sauté mode and add in the kale. Stir until wilted, about 1-2 minutes.

Stir in the heavy cream and continue cooking until heated through, about 1 minute. Season with salt and pepper to taste, as needed. Remove from the heat.

Garnish with fresh grated parmesan and parsley and serve immediately.

Part 2

South Beach Diet Recipes

Rose Spritz

- Absolute: 5 min
- Dynamic: 5 min
- Yield: 1 beverage

Fixings

3 ounces pink prosecco
2 ounces seltzer
1 ounce harsh orange alcohol, for example, Aperol
1/2 ounce grapefruit juice
1 grapefruit bend
1 sprig new mint

Bearings

1.Fill a white wine glass most of the way with ice. Include the prosecco, seltzer, orange alcohol and grapefruit squeeze and mix. Enhancement with a grapefruit wind and a sprig of mint.

Sexx on the Beach

- All out: 3 min
- Prep: 3 min
- Yield: 1 serving

Fixings

1/2-ounce vodka (prescribed: Skyy Vodka)
1/2-ounce melon alcohol (prescribed: Midori Melon
    Liqueur)
1/2-ounce raspberry alcohol (prescribed: Chambord)
Sprinkle pineapple juice

Sprinkle cranberry juice

Headings
1.Empty all fixings into a mixed drink shaker loaded up
with ice. Shake and strain into a 14-ounce glass loaded
up with ice. Present with a tall straw.

Shoreline Pub Oysters Rockafellar

- Complete: 25 min
- Prep: 20 mi
- Cook: 5 min
- Yield: 4 to 6 servings

Fixings

4 tablespoons olive oil
1/3 cup newly hacked garlic
1 pound new child spinach
1 cup hacked newly cooked bacon
1/2 cup disintegrated feta cheddar
1/2 cup ground Parmesan, in addition to additional for
    sprinkling 1/4 cup overwhelming whipping cream
    18 half-shell shellfish

Bearings

1.   Preheat the oven.
2.   Warmth the olive oil in a medium pot over medium warmth. Include the garlic and mix 1 moment,

at that point include the spinach, blending always until the spinach has cooked (don't overcook!). Make a point to blend the garlic and don't give it a chance to consume on the base of the container.

3.   Spot the garlic and spinach in a strainer and let the fluid strain 1 to 2 minutes.

4.   Move to a blending bowl and include the bacon, feta, Parmesan and whipping cream and blend well. Spot 1 loading tablespoon of the blend onto each opened clam and sprinkle each with ground Parmesan. Spot under the grill until brilliant dark colored, around 2 minutes.

5.   Prepared to serve!

Cook's Note

Chesapeake Bay Eastern Shore clams function admirably! If not accessible, I propose Gulf of Mexico clams.

French Onion Soup

- All out: 1 hr 10 min
- Prep: 10 min
- Cook: 1 hr
- Yield: 4 to 6 servings

Fixings

2 1/2 pounds yellow onions, divided, and cut 1/4-inch
    thick (8 cups)
1/4 pound unsalted margarine
1 straight leaf
1/2 cup medium-dry sherry
1/2 cup liquor or Cognac
1/2 cups great dry white wine
4 cups hamburger stock
4 cups veal stock
1 tablespoon genuine salt
1/2 teaspoon crisply ground white pepper
Crisply ground Parmesan

Headings

1.In an enormous stockpot on medium-high heat, saute
the onions with the spread and inlet leaf for 20
minutes, until the onions turn a rich brilliant dark
colored shading. Deglaze the skillet with the sherry and
schnaps and stew revealed for 5 minutes. Include the
white wine and stew revealed for 15 additional
minutes.

2.Include the hamburger and veal stocks in addition to
salt and pepper. Heat to the point of boiling, at that
point stew revealed for 20 minutes. Evacuate the inlet
leaf, taste for salt and pepper, and serve hot with
ground Parmesan.

Barbecued Herb Shrimp

- All out: 18 min
- Prep: 15 min
- Cook: 3 min
- Yield: 6 servings

Fixings

2 pounds enormous shrimp (16 to 20 for every pound), stripped and deveined (see note)
3 cloves garlic, minced
1 medium yellow onion, little diced
1/4 cup minced crisp parsley
1/4 cup minced crisp basil
1 teaspoon dry mustard
2 teaspoons Dijon mustard
2 teaspoons fit salt
1/2 teaspoon naturally ground dark pepper
1/4 cup great olive oil
1 lemon, squeezed

Headings

1.Join every one of the fixings and enable them to marinate for 1 hour at room temperature or spread and refrigerate for as long as 2 days.

2.Stick the shrimp. I utilize 3 or 4 shrimp on a 12-inch stick for supper. Warmth a flame broil with coals and brush the barbecue with oil to keep the shrimp from staying. Flame broil the shrimp for just 1/2 minutes on each side.

Gazpacho

- All out: 20 min
- Prep: 20 min
- Yield: 4 to 6 servings

Fixings

1 nursery cucumber, divided and seeded, however not
   stripped
2 red ringer peppers, cored and seeded
4 plum tomatoes
1 red onion
3 garlic cloves, minced
23 ounces tomato juice (3 cups)
1/4 cup white wine vinegar
1/4 cup great olive oil
1/2 tablespoon genuine salt
1 teaspoons crisply ground dark pepper

Headings

1.Generally cleave the cucumbers, ringer peppers,
tomatoes, and red onions into 1-inch blocks. Put every
vegetable independently into a sustenance processor

fitted with a steel sharp edge and heartbeat until it is coarsely hacked. Don't overprocess!

2.After every vegetable is handled, consolidate them in an enormous bowl and include the garlic, tomato juice, vinegar, olive oil, salt, and pepper. Blend well and chill before serving. The more extended gazpacho sits, the more the flavors create.

Long Beach Coleslaw

- Absolute: 50 min
- Prep: 43 min
- Cook: 7 min
- Yield: 6 to 8 servings

Fixings

2 tablespoons extra-virgin olive oil
1/2 red onion, daintily cut
2 tablespoons minced garlic (around 6 cloves)
1/2 little head red cabbage, cut and cut into 1/8-inch shreds Fine ocean salt and newly ground pepper 1 cup red wine vinegar
2 heads chunk of ice lettuce, cut and cut into 1-inch squares
1 cup thick, stout blue cheddar plate of mixed greens dressing

Bearings

1.   In a huge skillet over medium-high heat, consolidate the olive oil, red onion and garlic and cook 2 minutes (don't dark colored). Include the cabbage, 1

teaspoon salt, 1 tablespoon pepper and the vinegar and blend altogether; cook 3 to 5 minutes, until the cabbage is delicate. Move to a bowl and let cool to room temperature, at that point refrigerate 30 minutes.

In an enormous plate of mixed greens bowl, hurl the lettuce with the blue cheddar dressing. Channel the cabbage and delicately blend with the chunk of ice and dressing. Add more pepper to taste. Serve right away.

Shoreline Blanket Clambake

- All out: 1hr
- Prep: 30 min
- Cook: 3 hr 30 min
- Yield: : 8 to 12 servings

Fixings

8 purple potatoes
8 ears corn
8 lobster tails
16 lobster paws
2 kielbasa, split and cut in 8 pieces

8 dozen hard-shell mollusks, for example, cherrystone or littleneck
2 entire struggles, enveloped by aluminum foil with thyme, oil, and lemon cuts
8 dozen shellfish

Bearings

1. Dive a shallow pit in the sand and line with enormous stones. Assemble driftwood from the shoreline and heap over the coals. Make a blaze by consuming the wood for 1 to 2 hours until the stones are super hot. Rack off the fiery debris. Set 1 ash obstruct on each edge of the pit to frame the base. Lay a grill grind (or a bit of steel) on top to make a table. Accumulate kelp from the shoreline and spot a thick layer on the metal.

2. Spot the potatoes and corn on the rack, at that point spread with a flimsy layer of ocean growth. Hill the lobster tails, hooks and kielbasa equally on top, at that point spread with another flimsy layer of ocean growth. Set the shellfishes and struggle on top and spread with another layer of ocean growth.

At long last, set the clams on top, at that point spread with a thick layer of kelp. The juice from the fish will dribble down and season the corn and potatoes. Spread the whole heat with burlap or a covering absorbed seawater. The canvas traps in the ocean growth steam and heats the nourishment. Keep the canvas wet by pouring seawater over the top if necessary. Cook until the mollusks open and the lobster is brilliant red, around 1 to 1/2 hours.

Shellfish Bake on the Beach

- All out: 3 hr 20 min
- Prep: 20 min
- Idle: 2 hr
- Cook: 1 hr
- Yield: 6 to 8 servings

Fixings

2 sticks (1/2 pound) unsalted margarine, mellowed
1/2 cup ground Parmesan, in addition to additional for topping
1/2 cup finely slashed blended herbs, for example, parsley, chives, and thyme
Fit salt and crisply ground dark pepper
4 pounds half and half potatoes
8 ears corn
4 pounds kielbasa, cut into pieces
8 dozen hard-shell shellfishes, for example, cherrystone or littleneck

Headings

1.   Delve a shallow pit in the sand and line it with huge stones. Heap wood over the coals. Consume the wood for 1 to 2 hours until the stones are scorching; rake off the slag. Set 1 soot hinder on each edge of the pit to frame the base; lay a grill grind on top to make a table.

2.   While the stones are warming set up the herb spread: Mix the margarine with the cheddar and herbs; season it with salt and pepper. Refrigerate until prepared to utilize.

3.   Spot a thick layer of kelp on the mesh. Spot a layer of potatoes on the rack and spread them with a dainty layer of ocean growth. Put the corn on straightaway and afterward another flimsy layer of ocean growth. Presently put on the kielbasa and top it with a meager layer of ocean growth. Next hill the shellfishes on top and spread with a thick layer of kelp. Spread the whole heat with burlap or a canvas absorbed ocean water. Keep the canvas wet by pouring ocean water over the top if necessary. Cook until the mollusks open and the potatoes are delicate, around 60 minutes.

4.   Draw the husks once again from the corn and expel the silk. Brush liberally with the herb margarine and enhancement with ground Parmesan.

Orzo Salad

- All out: 40 min
- Prep: 10 min
- Idle: 20 min
- Cook: 10 min
- Yield: 6 servings

Fixings

4 cups chicken stock
1/2 cups orzo
1 (15-ounce) can garbanzo beans, depleted and flushed
1/2 cups red and yellow tear tomatoes or grape tomatoes, divided
3/4 cup finely cleaved red onion
1/2 cup cleaved new basil leaves
1/4 cup cleaved new mint leaves
Around 3/4 cup Red Wine Vinaigrette, formula pursues
Salt and crisply ground dark pepper
Red Wine Vinaigrette:
1/2 cup red wine vinegar
1/4 cup crisp lemon juice
2 teaspoons nectar
2 teaspoons salt
3/4 teaspoon naturally ground dark pepper
1 cup extra-virgin olive oil

Headings

1.   Empty the juices into a substantial huge pan. Spread the skillet and heat the stock to the point of boiling over high heat. Blend in the orzo. Spread mostly and cook until the orzo is delicate yet at the same time firm to the nibble, blending every now and again, around 7 minutes. Channel the orzo through a strainer. Move the orzo to an enormous wide bowl and hurl until the orzo cools somewhat. Put aside to cool totally.

2.   Hurl the orzo with the beans, tomatoes, onion, basil, mint, and enough vinaigrette to coat. Season the plate of mixed greens, to taste, with salt and pepper, and serve at room temperature.

☐   *Red Wine Vinaigrette:*

1.   Blend the vinegar, lemon juice, nectar, salt, and pepper in a blender. With the machine running, step by step mix in the oil. Season the vinaigrette, to taste, with increasingly salt and pepper, whenever wanted.

2.   Yield: 1 3/4 cups

Linguine with Shrimp Scampi

- Complete: 30 min
- Prep: 20 min
- Cook: 10 min
- Yield: 3 servings

Fixings

Vegetable oil

Legitimate salt

3/4 pound linguine

3 tablespoons unsalted spread

2 1/2 tablespoons great olive oil

1/2 tablespoons minced garlic (4 cloves)

1 pound huge shrimp (around 16 shrimp), stripped and deveined

1/4 teaspoon newly ground dark pepper

1/3 cup hacked new parsley leaves

1/2 lemon, get-up-and-go ground

1/4 cup newly pressed lemon juice (2 lemons)

1/4 lemon, meagerly cut into equal parts rounds

1/8 teaspoon hot red pepper drops

Headings

1.Sprinkle some oil in an enormous pot of bubbling salted water, include 1 tablespoon of salt and the linguine, and cook for 7 to 10 minutes, or as per the bearings on the bundle.

2.In the mean time, in another huge (12-inch), substantial bottomed container, dissolve the spread and olive oil over medium-low heat. Include the garlic. Saute for 1 moment. Be cautious, the garlic consumes effectively! Include the shrimp, 1/2 teaspoons of salt, and the pepper and saute until the shrimp have quite recently turned pink, around 5 minutes, blending regularly. Expel from the warmth, include the parsley, lemon get-up-and-go, lemon juice, lemon cuts, and red pepper drops. Hurl to join.

3.At the point when the pasta is done, channel the cooked linguine and after that set it back in the pot. Promptly include the shrimp and sauce, hurl well, and serve.

Key Lime Pie Martini

- Absolute: 35 min
- Prep: 5 min
- Dormant: 30 min
- Yield: 1 beverage

Fixings

Graham wafer scraps, for rimming the glass
2 lime wedges
6 tablespoons (3 ounces) vanilla seasoned vodka
1/4 cup (2 ounces) key lime alcohol (suggested: KeKe
    Beach Key Lime Liqueur)
2 tablespoons pineapple juice
2 tablespoons overwhelming cream
Ice 3D shapes

Bearings

1.Pour the graham wafer scraps in a shallow dish. Rub a
lime wedge around the edge of a martini glass and roll

the edge in the graham saltine morsels. Chill the glass for 30 minutes or until prepared to serve.

2.Consolidate the vanilla vodka, key lime alcohol, pineapple squeeze, and cream in a shaker. Fill the shaker half full with ice and shake until all around mixed. Fill arranged martini glass, decorate with a lime wedge and serve right away.

Panzanella

- Absolute: 55 min
- Prep: 15 min
- Dormant: 30 min
- Cook: 10 min
- Yield: 12 servings

Fixings

3 tablespoons great olive oil

1 little French bread or boule, cut into 1-inch 3D shapes
   (6 cups)

1 teaspoon genuine salt

2 huge, ready tomatoes, cut into 1-inch 3D shapes

1 nursery cucumber, unpeeled, seeded, and cut 1/2-
   inch thick

1 red chime pepper, seeded and cut into 1-inch 3D
   shapes

1 yellow chime pepper, seeded and cut into 1-inch 3D
   shapes 1/2 red onion, cut in 1/2 and daintily cut

20 huge basil leaves, coarsely cleaved

3 tablespoons tricks, depleted

For the vinaigrette:

1 teaspoon finely minced garlic
1/2 teaspoon Dijon mustard
3 tablespoons Champagne vinegar
1/2 cup great olive oil
1/2 teaspoon genuine salt
1/4 teaspoon crisply ground dark pepper

Bearings

1.Warmth the oil in a huge saute container. Include the bread and salt; cook over low to medium warmth, hurling as often as possible, for 10 minutes, or until pleasantly seared. Include more oil as required.

2.For the vinaigrette, whisk every one of the fixings together.

3.In an enormous bowl, blend the tomatoes, cucumber, red pepper, yellow pepper, red onion, basil, and escapades. Include the bread solid shapes and hurl with the vinaigrette. Season generously with salt and pepper. Serve, or enable the plate of mixed greens to sit for about 30 minutes for the flavors to mix.

Chicken Katsu

- All out: 1 hr 36 min
- Prep: 20 min
- Latent: 1 hr
- Cook: 16 min
- Yield: 6 servings

Fixings

3/4 cup Aloha shoyu (it's the best, the main truly)
2 tablespoons nectar
Squeeze red pepper drops (just as much as you would encourage your solitary goldfish)
1 tablespoon sesame oil
1 bundle chicken bosom cutlets (4 to 6 pieces)
   1 egg
2 tablespoons water
Garlic powder (ensure it's powder NOT garlic salt)
1/2 cup shelled nut oil (more in the event that you utilize an enormous griddle)
1 cup mochiko (rice flour)
1 bundle panko (Japanese bread morsels)
   Serving proposals: sunomono and potato-macintosh plate of mixed greens

Headings

1.   Join the shoyu, nectar, pepper pieces, and sesame oil in a zip-top pack and shake everything together. At that point include the chicken. Give the chicken a chance to marinate refrigerated medium-term, or possibly 60 minutes.

2.   Subsequent to marinating remove the chicken from the sack and get it dry with paper towels.

3.   Beat the egg, include the water and garlic powder, to taste. Try not to fear the garlic here, yet don't go vampire chasing either.

4.   Warmth the oil in a griddle over medium/medium-high heat. Make sure to watch the oil, in the event that it starts to smoke - turn it down a score.

5.   Dig the chicken in the rice flour, at that point egg, trailed by the panko. Spot the cutlet into the dish and fry for 5 to 8 minutes on each side. The panko ought to be fresh and brilliant dark colored. Spot on a drying rack and wrap up different pieces.

6.   I like to serve this with sunomono and potato-macintosh plate of mixed greens.

7.   This is effectively a 30 moment supper.

Panzanella

- Absolute: 55 min
- Prep: 15 min

- Dormant: 30 min
- Cook: 10 min
- Yield: 12 servings

Fixings

3 tablespoons great olive oil
1 little French bread or boule, cut into 1-inch 3D shapes (6 cups)
1 teaspoon genuine salt
2 huge, ready tomatoes, cut into 1-inch 3D shapes
1 nursery cucumber, unpeeled, seeded, and cut 1/2-inch thick
1 red chime pepper, seeded and cut into 1-inch 3D shapes
1 yellow chime pepper, seeded and cut into 1-inch 3D shapes 1/2 red onion, cut in 1/2 and daintily cut
20 huge basil leaves, coarsely cleaved
3 tablespoons tricks, depleted
For the vinaigrette:
1 teaspoon finely minced garlic
1/2 teaspoon Dijon mustard
3 tablespoons Champagne vinegar
1/2 cup great olive oil
1/2 teaspoon genuine salt
1/4 teaspoon crisply ground dark pepper

Bearings

1.   Warmth the oil in a huge saute container. Include the bread and salt; cook over low to medium warmth, hurling as often as possible, for 10 minutes, or until pleasantly seared. Include more oil as required.

2.   For the vinaigrette, whisk every one of the fixings together.

3.   In an enormous bowl, blend the tomatoes, cucumber, red pepper, yellow pepper, red onion, basil, and escapades. Include the bread solid shapes and hurl with the vinaigrette. Season generously with salt and pepper. Serve, or enable the plate of mixed greens to sit for about 30 minutes for the flavors to mix.

6 Hour Tri-tip Marinade

Absolute: 6 hr 50 min

Prep: 15 min

Dormant: 6 hr

Cook: 35 min

Yield: 6 to 8 servings

    Fixings

1 cup lemon juice
1 cup soybean oil

1/2 cup white sugar
1/2 cup soy sauce
1/2 cup dark pepper
1/2 cup garlic salt (suggested: Lawry's)
1/2 cup cleaved garlic
1/2 cup cleaved dried onions
Two 4-pound tri-tips, cut

Bearings

1.	To make the marinade, blend the majority of the fixings with the exception of the meat in a huge blending bowl. Spot the cut tri-tips in a plastic compartment and pour the marinade over. Give stand access the icebox for in any event 6 hours.

2.	Warmth barbecue to medium temperature.

3.	Spot tri-tips on barbecue at a 45-degree edge to set up flame broil checks and cook around 35 minutes, or until cooked to wanted doneness. Expel the tri-tips from the barbecue and let rest around 2 to 5 minutes before cutting. Present with your preferred side dishes.

Gazpacho

- All out: 20 min
- Prep: 20 min
- Yield: 4 to 6 servings

Fixings

1 nursery cucumber, divided and seeded, however not stripped
2 red ringer peppers, cored and seeded
4 plum tomatoes
1 red onion
3 garlic cloves, minced
23 ounces tomato juice (3 cups)
1/4 cup white wine vinegar
1/4 cup great olive oil
1/2 tablespoon genuine salt
1 teaspoons crisply ground dark pepper

Headings

1.Generally cleave the cucumbers, ringer peppers, tomatoes, and red onions into 1-inch blocks. Put every vegetable independently into a sustenance processor fitted with a steel sharp edge and heartbeat until it is coarsely hacked. Don't overprocess!

2.After every vegetable is handled, consolidate them in an enormous bowl and include the garlic, tomato juice, vinegar, olive oil, salt, and pepper. Blend well and chill before serving. The more extended gazpacho sits, the more the flavors create.

Panzanella

- Absolute: 55 min
- Prep: 15 min
- Dormant: 30 min
- Cook: 10 min
- Yield: 12 servings

Fixings

3 tablespoons great olive oil
1 little French bread or boule, cut into 1-inch 3D shapes (6 cups)
1 teaspoon genuine salt
2 huge, ready tomatoes, cut into 1-inch 3D shapes

1 nursery cucumber, unpeeled, seeded, and cut 1/2-inch thick
1 red chime pepper, seeded and cut into 1-inch 3D shapes
1 yellow chime pepper, seeded and cut into 1-inch 3D shapes 1/2 red onion, cut in 1/2 and daintily cut
20 huge basil leaves, coarsely cleaved
3 tablespoons tricks, depleted
For the vinaigrette:
1 teaspoon finely minced garlic
1/2 teaspoon Dijon mustard
3 tablespoons Champagne vinegar
1/2 cup great olive oil
1/2 teaspoon genuine salt
   1/4 teaspoon crisply ground dark pepper

Bearings

1.Warmth the oil in a huge saute container. Include the bread and salt; cook over low to medium warmth, hurling as often as possible, for 10 minutes, or until pleasantly seared. Include more oil as required.

2.For the vinaigrette, whisk every one of the fixings together.
3.In an enormous bowl, blend the tomatoes, cucumber, red pepper, yellow pepper, red onion, basil, and escapades. Include the bread solid shapes and hurl with the vinaigrette. Season generously with salt and pepper. Serve, or enable the plate of mixed greens to sit for about 30 minutes for the flavors to mix.

Sacripantina

Fixings

For the meringues:

6 enormous egg whites, at room temperature
1/8 teaspoon cream of tartar
2 cups sugar
1 teaspoon amaretto
2 teaspoons white vinegar
For the Genovese Butter Cake:
7 enormous eggs
3 enormous egg yolks
1 cup sugar
1/2 cups universally handy flour
1/2 teaspoon heating powder
13 tablespoons unsalted margarine, dissolved

For the Zabaglione Filling:

8 enormous egg yolks
1/3 cup cream sherry
1/2 cup sugar
Finely ground pizzazz of 1 orange
1 sheet gelatin (9 by 2 1/2 inches) or 1 teaspoon
powdered gelatin 1 cup substantial cream, whipped

to medium-delicate pinnacles For the Cream Frosting:

1 cup substantial cream

2 tablespoons sugar

1 teaspoon vanilla concentrate

1 tablespoon cognac

For the Simple Syrup:

1/2 cup sugar

1/4 cup cream sherry

For Assembly:

1 cup amaretti treat pieces

Cocoa powder for cleaning

Bearings

1.For the meringues: Preheat the stove to 200 to 250 degrees fahrenheit. Line a heating sheet with material.

2.In a huge bowl, beat the egg whites with an electric blender until foamy. Include the cream of tartar and keep beating until delicate pinnacles structure. Lower the speed and bit by bit beat in the sugar. Include the amaretto and vinegar and beat at medium speed until firm, shiny pinnacles structure, around 8 minutes longer. Utilizing a huge kitchen spoon and your scarcely sodden fingers, shape the meringue into twelve 4x3-inch ovals on the material lined heating sheet.

3.Spot on the most minimal rack in the broiler and prepare for around 45 minutes, until brilliant darker. Cool on wire racks. Store in a firmly shut plastic holder at room temperature.

4.For the Genovese Butter Cake: Preheat the broiler to 350 degrees fahrenheit. Spread and flour a 8-inch springform skillet.

5.In a huge metal bowl, beat the eggs, yolks and sugar with an electric blender on fast until significantly increased in volume, around 7 minutes.

6.Spot the bowl over a pot of water, carry the water to a stew, and rush for 1 to 2 minutes to warm the eggs somewhat. Expel from the warmth.

7.Filter the flour and heating powder together and overlay into the egg blend. Move one-eighth of the player to a little bowl and whisk the softened margarine into it. Empty the cake hitter into the readied cake container.

8.Heat for 1 to 1/4 hours, or until a wooden stick embedded into the middle confesses all. Expel from the broiler and cool totally on a wire rack. (The cake can be made multi day ahead if firmly enveloped by plastic.)

9.For the Zabaglione Filling: Make a water shower by filling a huge profound pot half-full with water. Consolidate the yolks, cream sherry, sugar and orange pizzazz in an enormous bowl (ideally copper, to get more volume). Spot the bowl over the water and, while whisking the eggs overwhelmingly, carry the water to a stew over medium-low heat. Keep racing for around 5 minutes, or until the blend thickens and is light and cushioned. Expel the bowl from the warmth and let cool. (Leave the water shower over low heat.)

10.Spot the gelatin sheet, if utilizing, in virus water to mellow. Whenever delicate, press out the abundance water, at that point race into the egg blend. Or then again, for powdered gelatin, put 2 tablespoons cold water in a little dish and sprinkle the gelatin over the water. Let represent 1 moment to mellow, at that point rush into the egg blend. Return the bowl of egg blend to the stewing water shower and whisk continually over medium-low heat until the gelatin is completely disintegrated, around 2 minutes. Be mindful so as not to overcook the eggs, as they may turn sour, and ensure when racing to bring the majority of the blend up from the base of the bowl. Refrigerate until cold, whisking every so often, at that point crease in the whipped cream.

11.For the Cream Frosting: In a medium bowl whip the cream with the sugar, vanilla, and liquor to hardened pinnacles. Put aside in the fridge.

12.For the Simple Syrup: Over medium warmth, break down the sugar in 1/4 cup water and the sherry.

13.To Assemble: Place the cake on a cake stand. With a long sharp blade, trim off the extremely top (around

107

1/8 inch) of the cake. To cut the cake into 3 equivalent rounds, score 2 equitably dispersed lines all around the sides of the cake. Cut into the score lines around 1 inch right around the cake, at that point make a well put together completely through the cake to isolate it into three layers. With a sharp blade, trim off the external dark colored edges of each layer.

14. Spot the top layer of cake on a level serving plate. Spot the cake ring around the cake. Plunge a baked good brush into the straightforward syrup and brush it liberally onto the cake layer to dampen it. Spread about portion of the zabaglione on top. Include the following layer of cake, brush with the syrup, and top with the rest of the syrup and refrigerate for in any event 30 minutes, or medium-term, to set.

15. Expel the ring from the cake. Ice the entire cake with the cream icing, spreading it in all respects equitably and easily. (Utilize a cake brush on the off chance that you have one.) Sprinkle the amaretti morsels on top. Residue the highest points of the meringues with cocoa, at that point press them the long way into the sides of the cake, dispersing them equitably. Serve quickly, or refrigerate until prepared to serve, or medium-term.

Key Lime Pie Martini

- Absolute: 35 min

- Prep: 5 min

- Dormant: 30 min

- Yield: 1 beverage

Fixings

Graham wafer scraps, for rimming the glass
2 lime wedges
6 tablespoons (3 ounces) vanilla seasoned vodka
1/4 cup (2 ounces) key lime alcohol (suggested: KeKe Beach Key Lime Liqueur)
2 tablespoons pineapple juice
2 tablespoons overwhelming cream
Ice 3D shapes

Bearings

1.Pour the graham wafer scraps in a shallow dish. Rub a lime wedge around the edge of a martini glass and roll the edge in the graham saltine morsels. Chill the glass for 30 minutes or until prepared to serve.

2.Consolidate the vanilla vodka, key lime alcohol, pineapple squeeze, and cream in a shaker. Fill the shaker half full with ice and shake until all around mixed. Fill arranged martini glass, decorate with a lime wedge and serve right away.

Sexx on the Beach

- All out: 3 min

- Prep: 3 min

- Yield: 1 serving

Fixings

1/2-ounce vodka (prescribed: Skyy Vodka)

1/2-ounce melon alcohol (prescribed: Midori Melon Liqueur)

1/2-ounce raspberry alcohol (prescribed: Chambord)

Sprinkle pineapple juice

Sprinkle cranberry juice

Headings

1.Empty all fixings into a mixed drink shaker loaded up with ice. Shake and strain into a 14-ounce glass loaded up with ice. Present with a tall straw.

Barbecued Herb Shrimp

- All out: 18 min

- Prep: 15 min

- Cook: 3 min

- Yield: 6 servings

Fixings

2 pounds enormous shrimp (16 to 20 for every pound), stripped and deveined (see note)

3 cloves garlic, minced

1 medium yellow onion, little diced

1/4 cup minced crisp parsley

1/4 cup minced crisp basil

1 teaspoon dry mustard

2 teaspoons Dijon mustard

2 teaspoons fit salt

1/2 teaspoon naturally ground dark pepper

1/4 cup great olive oil

1 lemon, squeezed

Headings

1.Join every one of the fixings and enable them to marinate for 1 hour at room temperature or spread and refrigerate for as long as 2 days.

2.Stick the shrimp. I utilize 3 or 4 shrimp on a 12-inch stick for supper. Warmth a flame broil with coals and brush the barbecue with oil to keep the shrimp from staying. Flame broil the shrimp for just 1/2 minutes on each side.

Cook's Note

I leave the tails on when I'm stripping the shrimp.

Salmon with Lemon, Capers, and Rosemary

- Complete: 30 min

- Prep: 20 min

- Cook: 10 min

- Yield: 4 servings

Fixings

4 (6-ounce) salmon filets
1/4 cup extra-virgin olive oil
1/2 teaspoon salt
1/2 teaspoon newly ground dark pepper
1 tablespoon minced new rosemary leaves
8 lemon cuts (around 2 lemons)
1/4 cup lemon juice (around 1 lemon)
1/2 cup Marsala wine (or white wine)
4 teaspoons tricks
    4 bits of aluminum foil

Bearings

1.Brush top and base of salmon filets with olive oil and season with salt, pepper, and rosemary. Spot each bit of prepared salmon on a bit of foil huge enough to overlap over and seal. Top the each bit of salmon with 2 lemon cuts, 1 tablespoon of lemon juice, 2 tablespoons of wine, and 1 teaspoon of tricks. Wrap up salmon firmly in the foil bundles.

2.Spot a flame broil skillet over medium-high heat or preheat a gas or charcoal barbecue. Spot the foil bundles on the hot flame broil and cook for 10 minutes for a 1-inch thick bit of salmon. Serve in the foil bundles.

Grilled Chicken

- All out: 3 hr 50 min
- Prep: 5 min
- Idle: 3 hr
- Cook: 45 min

Yield: 6 servings

Fixings

2 chickens (2 1/2 to 3 pounds each), quartered, with backs evacuated

1 formula Barbecue Sauce, formula pursues
Grill Sauce:
1/2 cups hacked yellow onion (1 huge onion)
1 tablespoon minced garlic (3 cloves)
1/2 cup vegetable oil
1 cup tomato glue (10 ounces)
1 cup juice vinegar

1 cup nectar
1/2 cup Worcestershire sauce
1 cup Dijon mustard
1/2 cup soy sauce
1 cup hoisin sauce
2 tablespoons stew powder
1 tablespoon ground cumin
1/2 tablespoon squashed red pepper chips

Bearings

1.Marinate the chickens in 2/3 of the grill sauce for a couple of hours or medium-term in the icebox.

2.Warmth the coals in a charcoal barbecue. Spread the base of the barbecue with a solitary layer of hot coals and after that include a couple of more coals 5 minutes before cooking, which will prop the flame up longer. Spot the chicken quarters on the barbecue, skin side down, and cook for around 45 minutes, turning a few times to cook equally on the two sides. Brush with the marinade as required. The chicken quarters are done when you embed a blade between a leg and thigh and the juices run clear. Dispose of any unused marinade.

3.Present with additional grill sauce as an afterthought.

Grill Sauce:

1.In a huge pot on low heat, saute the onions and garlic with the vegetable oil for 10 to 15 minutes, until the onions are translucent however not seared. Include the tomato glue, vinegar, nectar, Worcestershire sauce, mustard, soy sauce, hoisin sauce, bean stew powder, cumin, and red pepper pieces. Stew revealed on low heat for 30 minutes. Use promptly or store in the icebox.

2.Yield: 1/2 quarts

Red Bean Beach Salad

- All out: 1 hr 20 min
- Prep: 20 min

- Idle: 1 hr
- Yield: 4 to 6 servings

Fixings

2 (15-ounce) jars red kidney beans, depleted and flushed
2 celery stalks, meagerly cut
1 enormous ready tomato, cored, divided and cleaved
1/2 cup cleaved sweet pickles
1/2 little red or yellow onion, finely minced
1/2 cup extra-virgin olive oil
1/4 cup juice vinegar
1 teaspoon Worcestershire sauce
1 teaspoon sugar
1/2 teaspoon ground cloves
1/2 teaspoon sweet paprika
   Salt
Crisply ground dark pepper
   1 teaspoon finely cleaved crisp oregano leaves

Headings

1.Blend the beans, celery, tomatoes, pickles, and onion together in an enormous bowl. In a little bowl, whisk the olive oil, vinegar, Worcestershire sauce, sugar, cloves, paprika, salt and pepper. Pour the serving of mixed greens dressing over the beans and hurl to coat. Spread with cling wrap and refrigerate for in any event 1 hour or medium-term before serving.

Long Beach Coleslaw

- All out: 17 min
- Prep: 10 min
- Cook: 7 min
- Yield: 6 to 8 servings

Fixings

2 tablespoons extra-virgin olive oil
1/2 red onion, meagerly cut
2 tablespoons garlic, minced
1/2 little head red cabbage, cleaned and cut into 1/8-inch, julienned 1 tablespoon crisply ground dark pepper 1 teaspoon ocean salt
8 ounces red wine vinegar
2 Iceberg lettuce heads, cleaned and cut into 1-inch pieces
12-ounces blue cheddar dressing, thick and stout

Headings

1.In medium saute skillet over medium warmth, include olive oil, onion and garlic, cook for 2 minutes, don't let dark colored. Include cabbage, pepper, salt, and vinegar. Blend altogether, and cook for 3 to 5 minutes until cabbage is delicate. Expel to a bowl and let chill in cooler until cool.

2.In enormous plate of mixed greens bowl, include Iceberg lettuce and hurl with blue cheddar dressing.

3.Strain cabbage blend of any fluid and daintily blend with Iceberg and blue cheddar dressing. Include pepper, to taste.

Filet of Beef Sandwiches

- Complete: 15 min
- Prep: 15 min
- Yield: 4 sandwiches

Fixings

1/4 pound blue d'Auvergne or other smooth blue cheddar
2/3 cup sharp cream
1/3 cup mayonnaise
1/2 teaspoons Worcestershire sauce
1 teaspoon legitimate salt
1 teaspoon newly ground dark pepper

To gather:

1 portion wellbeing or 7-grain bread
1/2 pounds uncommon filet of meat meagerly cut, formula pursues
1 pack arugula

Legitimate salt
Newly ground dark pepper
2 tablespoons unsalted spread, at room temperature

Filet of Beef:

1/2 pounds entire filet of meat cut and tied
2 tablespoons dissolved margarine
1 tablespoon salt
1 tablespoon coarsely ground dark pepper

Bearings

1.For the dressing, crush the blue cheddar with a fork and mix with the harsh cream, mayonnaise, Worcestershire sauce, salt, and pepper.

2.To make the sandwiches, cut the bread into 8 cuts, each cut 1/4 inch thick. Spread 4 of the cuts thickly with the dressing. Top with cuts of meat and arugula and sprinkle with salt and pepper. Spread the remainder of the cuts of bread in all respects gently with margarine and spot, spread side down, over the meat.

Filet of Beef:

1.Preheat broiler 500 degrees F.

2.Liquefy 2 tablespoons of unsalted spread.

3.Spot hamburger on a preparing sheet and pat the outside dry with a paper towel. Utilizing a cake brush coat the meat with the softened margarine. Sprinkle equally with salt and pepper. Broil for 25 minutes at 500 degrees F for medium uncommon.

4.Expel the meat from the broiler, spread firmly with aluminum foil, and permit to rest at room temperature for 20 minutes before cutting.

Niman Ranch Burgers

- Absolute: 1 hr 10 min
- Prep: 20 min
- Cook: 50 min
- Yield: 6 servings

Fixings

2 pounds ground Niman Ranch meat or different grass-sustained premium hamburger (80 percent lean and 20 percent fat)
1 tablespoon great Dijon mustard
3 tablespoons great olive oil, in addition to extra for brushing the flame broil
1 teaspoon legitimate salt
1 teaspoon newly ground dark pepper
3 sandwich-size English biscuits, split
Great mayonnaise
    Caramelized Onions, formula pursues

Caramelized Onions:

2 tablespoons great olive oil
2 tablespoons unsalted spread

2 pounds yellow onions, stripped and cut down the middle rounds 1/2 teaspoon crisp thyme leaves
2 tablespoons sherry wine vinegar
1 teaspoon genuine salt
    1/2 teaspoon crisply ground dark pepper

Headings

1.Fabricate a charcoal flame or warmth a gas barbecue.

2.Spot the ground hamburger in a huge bowl and include the mustard, olive oil, salt, and pepper. Blend tenderly with a fork to consolidate, taking consideration not to pack the fixings. Shape the meat into 6 (3 1/2-inch) patties of equivalent size and thickness.

3.At the point when the flame broil is medium-hot, brush the barbecue grind with oil to shield the burgers from staying. Spot the burgers on the barbecue and cook for 4 minutes. Utilizing a major spatula, turn the burgers and cook for another 3 to 4 minutes, until medium-uncommon or more, or cook longer on the off chance that you incline toward cheeseburgers all the more all around done.

4.Then, break separated the English biscuits and toast the 6 parts chop side down on the barbecue. Spread every half with mayonnaise and top with a burger and after that with a storing tablespoon of caramelized onions. Serve hot.

Caramelized Onions:

1.Warmth the olive oil and margarine in an enormous shallow pot, include the onions and thyme, and hurl with the oil. Spot the cover on top and cook over medium-low heat for around 10 minutes to sweat the onions. Evacuate the cover and keep on cooking over medium-low heat, mixing at times, for 25 to 30 minutes, until the onions are caramelized and brilliant dark colored. On the off chance that the onions are cooking excessively quick, bring down the warmth. Include the vinegar, salt, and pepper and cook for 2 additional minutes, scratching the dark colored bits from the dish. Season to taste (they ought to be in all respects exceptionally prepared).

Flame broiled Skirt Steak with Sweet Roasted Tomato Sauce and Roasted Shrimp, Black Bean and Orzo Salad

- Absolute: 2 hr 5 min
- Prep: 30 min

- Idle: 1 hr
- Cook: 35 min
- Yield: 4 to 6 servings

Fixings

Steak:

1 skirt steak (around 2 pounds)
Salt and ground dark pepper
1 cup crisp squeezed orange
1/4 cup extra-virgin olive oil
1/4 cup slashed crisp cilantro
1/4 cup slashed crisp parsley
1/2 teaspoon ground cumin
1 clove garlic

Tomato Sauce:

1 16 ounces sweet grape tomatoes
2 cloves garlic
1 serrano chile pepper, divided
2 tablespoons extra-virgin olive oil
1 teaspoon salt
1/2 teaspoon ground dark pepper
1/4 teaspoon ground cumin
1/4 cup chicken stock
1 teaspoon agave nectar
Serving of mixed greens:
1/2 pounds shrimp, 31/40 size, stripped and deveined

1/4 cup extra-virgin olive oil

Salt and ground dark pepper

2 cups canned dark beans, depleted and flushed

2 cups slashed cucumber

2 cups slashed red onion

2 cups slashed red ringer pepper

8 ounces disintegrated feta

1 cup slashed crisp parsley

1 cup slashed crisp cilantro

1 cup crisp crushed lime juice

1/2 cup slashed poblano chile pepper

1 serrano chile pepper, minced with seeds

2 cloves garlic, minced

8 ounces orzo, cooked to still somewhat firm

Headings

1.For the steak: Sprinkle the skirt steak with salt and pepper.

2.In a blender, include the squeezed orange, oil, cilantro, parsley, cumin and garlic and puree until smooth. Move the marinade to an enormous re-sealable plastic pack and include the steak. Seal the sack and shake delicately to coat the steak. Marinate the steak in the ice chest for 60 minutes. Carry the steak to room temp before flame broiling.

3.For the tomato sauce: Preheat the stove to 400 degrees F. On a preparing sheet, hurl the tomatoes, garlic and serrano with 1 tablespoon olive oil, salt, pepper and cumin. Broil in the broiler for 10 minutes. Move to a blender and mix with the chicken stock.

4. Warmth the staying 1 tablespoon olive oil in a pot over low warmth and include the sauce from the blender. Include the agave and stew for 5 minutes. Expel from the warmth and put in a safe spot.

5. For the serving of mixed greens: Spread the shrimp out on a heating sheet and shower with 2 tablespoons olive oil and sprinkle with salt and pepper. Broil the shrimp in the stove until cooked through, 10 to 12 minutes. Put in a safe spot and let cool.

6. Join the beans, cucumber, onions, chime pepper, feta, parsley, cilantro, lime juice, poblano, serrano and garlic in a huge bowl and hurl to consolidate. Include the shrimp, orzo and the staying 2 tablespoons olive oil. Blend together, taste and season with salt and pepper.

7. To complete: Preheat a flame broil or barbecue container to medium-high warmth and barbecue the steak 4 to 5 minutes on each side for medium/medium-uncommon. Let rest, and after that cut the steak and serve over the plate of mixed greens bested with tomato sauce.

8. Cook's Note: If making this dish for kids, you can constrain the warmth by substituting diced carrots for serrano chile peppers in the tomato sauce and the serving of mixed greens.

Flame broiled Whole Long Island Sound Porgy

- Complete: 15 min
- Prep: 5 min
- Cook: 10 min

Fixings

6 1/4 pounds Porgy
1 cup Extra Virgin Olive Oil
4 cloves squashed garlic
Salt and pepper to taste
1 lemon squeeze as it were
   1 tablespoon oregano

Bearings

1.Scale and gut new 1/4-11/2 pounds Porgy. Set up a charwood fire and enable the coals to torch to a hot white fiery debris. Brush the Porgy with olive oil (additional virgin) that has squashed garlic cloves blended in. Season with ocean salt and new processed pepper. Cook 2 1/2 minutes on each side ; evacuate. Shower all the more additional virgin olive oil over each fish ; press lemon. Sprinkle with dry Greek oregano.

Ribs with Big Daddy Rub

- All out: 2 hr 55 min
- Prep: 5 min
- Idle: 30 min
- Cook: 2 hr 20 min
- Yield: 4 to 6 servings

Fixings

5 pounds St. Louis style ribs
2 cups Big Daddy Rub, formula pursues
2 liters cola (prescribed: Coca-Cola)
4 cups water
   Apple Cider Buttermilk Dipping Sauce, formula pursues

Huge Daddy Rub:

3 cups darker sugar
1/4 cup fit salt
1/4 cup smoked paprika
2 tablespoons ground cumin
2 tablespoons hot bean stew powder

2 tablespoons cayenne

2 tablespoons naturally ground dark pepper

2 tablespoons red pepper drops

Apple Cider Buttermilk Dipping Sauce:

2 cups apple juice

1/4 cup granulated sugar

1 tablespoon red pepper drops

2 tablespoons buttermilk

1 teaspoon lemon juice

1 teaspoon lemon pizzazz

Headings

1.Preheat broiler to 350 degrees F.

2.Rub ribs with 1 cup Big Daddy Rub until equitably covered on the two sides. Enable ribs to marinate at room temperature for 30 minutes.

3.Spot ribs in 2 huge simmering container and spread with the cola and water. Spread with foil and cook in broiler for 1/2 hours. Expel ribs from stove and permit to cool. Cut ribs into individual-size pieces.

4.Preheat flame broil over medium-high heat.

5.Spot ribs on the flame broil. Brush on apple juice buttermilk sauce. Cook for extra 5 minutes.

6.In an enormous bowl, hurl ribs with another 1 cup of rub until very much covered. Spread ribs out on a sheet plate and prepare in the stove for an extra 20 minutes until caramelized.

7.Serve close by Apple Cider Buttermilk Sauce, chipotle aioli, or harissa rouille.

Huge Daddy Rub:

1.In a medium estimated bowl, blend all fixings until very much consolidated. Apple Cider Buttermilk Dipping Sauce:

2.In a medium pot include apple juice, sugar and red pepper on medium high heat. Decrease considerably. Empty blend into a different bowl. Include buttermilk. Blend completely and include lemon squeeze and pizzazz.

Mega Egga Macaroni Salad

- All out: 35 min
- Prep: 15 min
- Cook: 20 min
- Yield: 4 to 6 servings

Fixings

2 pounds elbow noodles
12 hard bubbled eggs, stripped and diced
1/2 onion, finely diced
4 celery stalks, finely diced
1/4 cup pickle relish
3 cups substantial mayonnaise
2 tablespoons salt, or to taste
1 teaspoon coarsely split dark pepper
Dash hot sauce
    1 tablespoon Worcestershire sauce

Headings

1.In an enormous pot with salt, bubble pasta for 12 to 15 minutes until cooked. Mix regularly. Channel and cool. Refrigerate for 30 minutes.

2.In an enormous pot with a dash of salt, include eggs medium high heat. Heat to the point of boiling. Spread and expel from warmth. Give eggs a chance to sit for 6 to 7 minutes. Evacuate eggs and stun in ice water. Once altogether cooled, strip eggs and generally dice.

3.Spot pasta in a huge bowl. Include onions, celery, eggs, relish, mayonnaise, salt and pepper, hot sauce and Worcestershire. Blend until all around consolidated.

Ahi Poke

- Complete: 15 min
- Prep: 15 min
    - Yield: 4 servings

Fixings

4 cups ahi, minced
1/2 cup onion, minced
1/4 cup green onion, minced
1 cup soy sauce
2 tablespoons sesame oil
3 tablespoons white truffle oil
1/2 tablespoon sambal olek
Hawaiian salt to taste
   1 teaspoon dark pepper

Bearings

1.Season ahi with Hawaiian salt. Include all fixings, blend well at that point chill.

Barbecued Halibut with Olive Bagna Caud

- All out: 30 min
- Dynamic: 30 min

- Yield: 4 servings

Fixings

Sauce:

1/4 cup olive oil
4 tablespoons (1/2 stick) unsalted margarine
2 teaspoons anchovy glue
2 cloves garlic, crushed and stripped
1/3 cup set blended olives, slashed
1/4 cup tear tomatoes, divided
    2 tablespoons slashed new Italian parsley

Fish:

Four 6-ounce skinless halibut filets
1 teaspoon fit salt
    2 teaspoons olive oil

Headings

1.Preheat a barbecue or flame broil skillet to medium high.

2.For the sauce: Put the olive oil, margarine, anchovy glue, garlic and olives in a little skillet. Warm over medium warmth until the spread is softened and the sauce is tenderly stewing, around 5 minutes. Expel from the warmth and mix in the tomatoes and parsley.

3.For the fish: Sprinkle the halibut filets on the two sides with the salt and shower with the olive oil. Flame broil until barbecue checked and obscure all through, around 4 minutes for every side.

4.Move the fish to a serving platter and spoon the bagna cauda over the top.

Flame broiled Clams with Basil Breadcrumbs

- Absolute: 30 min
- Prep: 25 min
- Cook: 5 min
- Yield: 6 servings

Fixings

1/2 cups coarse bread pieces, toasted
2 cloves garlic, minced
3 tablespoons great olive oil
2 tablespoons new lemon juice
6 sun-dried tomato parts in oil, depleted and coarsely hacked 1/2 cup hacked crisp basil leaves 1/4 cup toasted pine nuts
3/4 teaspoon legitimate salt
1/4 teaspoon newly ground dark pepper
24 littleneck mollusks, thoroughly cleaned
2 1/2 tablespoons dissolved margarine

Bearings

1.Warmth a gas flame broil or set up a charcoal barbecue with hot coals.

2.Consolidate the bread morsels, garlic, olive oil, lemon juice, sun-dried tomatoes, basil, pine nuts, salt and pepper in an enormous serving bowl and put in a safe spot.

3.At the point when the flame broil is hot, place the mollusks in 1 layer on the hot mesh and enable the warmth to open the shellfishes. They'll open bit by bit for around 5 minutes, at that point pop-open wide when they're set. Utilizing tongs, expel the mollusks from the barbecue and spot them in the bowl with the bread morsel blend and hurl together. Sprinkle with the dissolved spread, and serve hot.

Summer Succotash

- All out: 1 hr 20 min (incorporates sitting time)
- Dynamic: 20 min
- Yield: 4 to 6 servings

Fixings

8 ounces green beans or wax beans, cut, split and whitened Pieces from 3 ears of corn (around 2 1/2 cups)

1 cup cherry tomatoes (ideally Sungold), split
1 little red chime pepper, cut into strips
1/4 cup new mint leaves, slashed
2 tablespoons new oregano leaves, slashed
2 tablespoons white balsamic vinegar
1/4 cup extra-virgin olive oil
3/4 teaspoon legitimate salt
   One 8-ounce ball new mozzarella, diced

Bearings

1.Consolidate the green beans, corn parts, tomatoes, peppers, mint and oregano in a huge bowl and blend well. Include the vinegar, olive oil and salt and hurl to coat. Let sit for 1 hour to enable the flavors to wed. Overlap in the cheddar just before serving.

Mai Tai

- All out: 5 min
- Prep: 5 min
- Yield: 2 servings

Fixings

1 egg white, softly beaten*
  Sugar
1/2 cup white rum
1/4 cup Triple Sec
1/4 cup crisp squeezed orange
1/4 cup crisp lime juice
  Squashed ice

To improve:

Mixed drink fruits
Pineapple shapes
  Orange cuts

Headings

1.Plunge the edge of tall glasses into the egg whites, and after that the sugar. Put the rum, Triple Sec, and juices into a mixed drink shaker. Shake to blend. Fill the glasses with the ice and pour the mixed drink over it. Embellish with fruits, pineapple, or potentially orange cuts, and drink with a straw.

Flame broiled Beans with Parmesan

- Absolute: 10 min
- Dynamic: 10 min
- Yield: 4 servings

Fixings

1 pound blended green beans, for example, string, Romano and snow peas
2 tablespoons olive oil
1/2 teaspoon genuine salt
1/2 cup crisply ground Parmesan
    1/2 teaspoon lemon get-up-and-go

Bearings

1.Preheat a flame broil dish to medium high.

2.In a medium bowl, hurl the beans with the olive oil and salt. Flame broil the beans until brilliant green, delicate and marginally burned, 2 to 3 minutes for every side. Spot the flame broiled beans back in the bowl and hurl with the Parmesan and lemon pizzazz. Serve warm or at room temperature.

Kalua Pork

- Absolute: 4 hr 20 min
- Prep: 20 min
- Cook: 4 hr

- Yield: 4 to 6 servings

Fixings

- 8 pounds pork butt
- 4 tablespoons Hawaiian salt, partitioned
- 4 tablespoons in addition to a couple of drops fluid smoke, isolated
- 8 to 12 enormous ti leaves, ribs evacuated
- 2 cups bubbling water

Headings

1.Preheat broiler to 350 degrees F.

2.Subsequent to scoring pork on all sides with 1/4-inch cuts around 1-inch separated, rub with 3 tablespoons salt, at that point fluid smoke. Wrap the pork totally in ti leaves, tie with string, and envelop by foil. Spot meat in a shallow simmering dish with 2 cups of water and meal for 4 hours. Disintegrate 1 tablespoon Hawaiian salt in 2 cups bubbling water and include a couple of drops of fluid smoke. Shred the cooked pork and let remain in this answer for a couple of minutes before serving.

Lemon-Ricotta Pancakes

- All out: 45 min (incorporates sitting time)
- Dynamic: 30 min
  - Yield: 16 hotcakes

Fixings

2/3 cup universally handy flour

1/3 cup polenta

1 teaspoon heating powder

1/4 teaspoon genuine salt

1 cup buttermilk

1/2 cup part-skim ricotta cheddar, for example, Calabro

2 teaspoons ground lemon pizzazz (2 lemons)

2 eggs

Grapeseed oil

Maple syrup, warmed, for serving

Headings

1.In an enormous bowl, whisk together the flour, polenta, preparing powder and salt. In a huge estimating cup, whisk together the buttermilk, ricotta, lemon get-up-and-go and eggs. Pour the fluid fixings over the dry fixings and overlap together, utilizing an elastic spatula, until simply joined. Let sit for 15 minutes to enable the polenta to relax.

2.Preheat a rimmed frying pan to medium-low warm. Add oil to coat the iron.

3.With a 1/4-cup measure, scoop hitter onto the frying pan. Cook for 2 to 3 minutes for each side, until brilliant darker and cooked through. Evacuate the flapjacks to a plate and proceed with the rest of the hitter. Serve warm with bunches of warm maple syrup.

Goat Cheese Tart

- Absolute: 41 hr 25 min
- Prep: 45 min
- Dormant: 40 hr
- Cook: 40 min
- Yield: 6 servings

Fixings

1/2 cups generally useful flour, in addition to additional for tidying the board Legitimate salt
13 tablespoons cold unsalted spread, separated
3 to 4 tablespoons ice water
3/4 cup cleaved shallots (3 to 4 shallots)
10 1/2 ounces garlic-and-herb delicate goat cheddar (prescribed: Montrachet}
1 cup substantial cream
3 extra-enormous eggs
1/4 cup cleaved basil leaves
1/8 teaspoon crisply ground dark pepper

Headings

1.Preheat the broiler to 350 degrees F.

2.For the outside layer, put the flour and 1/4 teaspoon salt in the bowl of a sustenance processor fitted with the steel edge. Cut 12 tablespoons (1/2 sticks) of the margarine into huge shakers, add to the bowl, and heartbeat until the spread is the size of peas. With the machine running, include the ice water at the same time and procedure until the mixture turns out to be brittle. Don't overprocess. Dump the mixture out on a floured board, assemble it freely into a ball, spread with cling wrap, and refrigerate for 30 minutes.

3.Roll the mixture on a well-floured board and fit it into a 9-inch tart skillet with a removable sides, rolling the stick over the top to remove the overabundance batter. Margarine 1 side of a square of aluminum foil and fit it, spread side down, into the tart skillet. Fill the foil with rice or beans. Heat for 20 minutes. Expel the beans and foil from the tart shell, prick the base done with a fork, and prepare for an additional 10 minutes.

4.In the interim, heat the rest of the tablespoon of spread in a little skillet and saute the shallots over low heat for 5 minutes, or until delicate. Spot the goat cheddar in the bowl of the sustenance processor and procedure until brittle. Include the cream, eggs, basil, 1/4 teaspoon salt, and the pepper and procedure until mixed.

5.Disperse the cooked shallots over the base of the tart shell. Pour the goat cheddar blend over the shallots to fill the shell (if the shell has contracted, there might be extra filling). Prepare for 30 to 40 minutes, until the tart is firm when shaken and the top is delicately carmelized. Permit to cool for 10 minutes and serve hot or at room temperature.

Solidified S'mores

- All out: 2 hr 20 min (incorporates solidifying time)
- Dynamic: 20 min
- Yield: 10 s'mores

Fixings

Nonstick cooking shower
2 cups smaller than expected marshmallows
1 16 ounces vanilla frozen yogurt
1/2 cup smaller than expected chocolate chips
    10 entire graham saltines, broken fifty-fifty

Headings

1.Preheat the grill to high.

2.Shower a rimmed heating sheet with nonstick cooking splash. Spread the marshmallows on the preparing sheet and sear until profound darker, around 30 seconds. Expel from the broiler and put in a safe spot for 5 minutes to cool.

3.In a stand blender with the oar connection, beat the frozen yogurt on medium-low speed until simply delicate. Include the toasted marshmallows and the chocolate chips and blend on low until simply joined. Working rapidly, scoop around 3 tablespoons of the frozen yogurt blend onto half of the graham wafers. Top with the rest of the graham wafers and spot in the cooler. Stop until firm, at any rate 2 hours.

Cook's Note

In the event that the dessert blend is too delicate to even consider scooping onto the graham wafers, return the frozen yogurt to the cooler for 30 minutes to solidify marginally before continuing.

Key Lime Creme Brulee

- All out: 1 hr 15 min
- Prep: 1 hr
- Cook: 15 min
- Yield: 6 servings

Fixings

Filling:

3 egg yolks, in addition to 3 egg yolks
1/2 ounces sugar
10 ounces substantial cream
1 vanilla bean, split
2 ounces improved dense milk
    3 ounces key lime juice

Covering:

Puff baked good, locally acquired

Natural product puree, as an embellishment, discretionary

Bearings

1.Preheat stove to 350 degrees F.

2.Over a twofold kettle, whisk 3 egg yolks and sugar to a thick, strip like surface. In a different pot, consolidate the overwhelming cream and split vanilla bean, and heat to the point of boiling. Temper the egg yolk blend into the cream, by whisking a tad bit of the hot cream into the eggs, while continually whisking, and after that whisk the yolk blend again into the hot cream. Come back to the warmth and, while whisking consistently, complete the process of cooking to a custard organize, roughly 1 or 2 minutes.

3.For the second piece of the creme brulee, whisk the staying 3 egg yolks for 1 moment. Include the dense milk and rush for one more moment. Include the key lime squeeze step by step and race for 1 moment. Join the creme brulee loading up with the key lime filling and chill in the fridge until required.

4.To make the hull, reveal a sheet of puff cake slight, 20 by 10-inches. Cut 6 (4-inch breadth) hovers out of the puff cake to line 6 (3-inch) tart container. Give the mixture a chance to rest for 30 minutes in the fridge. Line the baked good rings with the cake batter and trim the abundance mixture flush to the edge of the ring. Spot a bit of material paper on every tart shell and load up with beans and prepare until brilliant, around 10 minutes. The shells ought to be extremely flimsy and even.

5.To gather, fill the shells with the key lime filling and level the tops with a spatula. Residue the highest points of the treats with sugar and utilizing a light caramelize the tops. Spot the treats on a plate and present with natural product puree, whenever wanted.

Burned Corn Guacamole with Corn Chips

- All out: 50 min
- Prep: 15 min
- Idle: 10 min
- Cook: 25 min
- Yield: 4 servings

Fixings

4 ears Perfectly Grilled Corn, formula pursues
4 tablespoons canola oil
Salt and naturally ground dark pepper
3 ready avocados, stripped, set and diced
1 serrano chile, finely diced
1 little red onion finely diced
1 lime, squeezed
1/4 cup slashed cilantro leaves
Blue, yellow and white corn chips, as backup
Flawlessly Grilled Corn:
4 ears corn
    Fit salt

Headings

1.Warmth the barbecue to high.

2.Expel the husks from the barbecued corn and dispose of. Brush the ears of corn with 2 tablespoons of the canola oil and season with salt and pepper. Flame broil the ears until the parts are gently brilliant dark colored on all sides, around 5 minutes. Expel the portions from the ears.

3.Spot the avocado in a medium bowl and pound somewhat with a fork. Include the corn, serrano, onion, lime juice, staying 2 tablespoons of oil, cilantro and salt and pepper and delicately blend to join. Present with fricasseed corn chips or warm flour tortillas.

Superbly Grilled Corn:

1.Warmth the flame broil to medium.

2.Force the external husks down the ear to the base. Strip away the silk from every ear of corn by hand. Crease husks once again into the right spot and tie the closures together with kitchen string. Spot the ears of corn in a huge bowl of virus water with 1 tablespoon of salt for 10 minutes.

3.Expel corn from water and shake off abundance. Spot the corn on the barbecue, close the spread and flame broil for 15 to 20 minutes, turning at regular intervals, or until portions are delicate when penetrated with a paring blade. Evacuate the husks and eat on the cob or expel the bits.

4.The most effective method to expel corn parts from cob: To expel bits from cobs of either crude or cooked corn, stand cob upstanding on its stem end in a huge dish, holding tip with fingers. Chop down the sides of cob with sharp paring blade, discharging bits without cutting into cob. Run dull edge of blade down the cob to discharge any residual corn and fluid.

Seared Couscous Salad

- Absolute: 58 min
- Prep: 10 min
- Dormant: 5 min
- Cook: 43 min
- Yield: 2 to 4 servings

Fixings

Couscous:

2 cups low-sodium chicken stock
1/2 teaspoon genuine salt
1 (10-ounce) box (1/4 cups) couscous (suggested: Near East)
1/4 cup extra-virgin olive oil

2 cloves garlic, stripped and squashed

4 ounces ricotta salata cheddar, cut into 1/2-inch pieces

1 little or 1/2 enormous cucumber, stripped, seeded, and cut into 1/2-inch pieces

1/4 cup sun-dried tomatoes, cleaved

1/4 cup ground Parmesan

1/4 cup cleaved crisp basil leaves

Dressing:

1/4 cup extra-virgin olive oil

Pizzazz and juice from 1/2 enormous lemon

1/2 teaspoon genuine salt

1/4 teaspoon crisply ground dark pepper

Headings

1.For the couscous: In a medium pan, heat the chicken juices and salt to the point of boiling over medium-high heat. Expel the skillet from the warmth and mix in the couscous. Spread until the fluid had been retained and the couscous is delicate, 5 to 6 minutes. Utilizing a fork, lighten the couscous and separate any knots.

2.In an enormous, nonstick skillet heat 1/4 cup oil over medium warmth. Include the garlic and cook until brilliant, 1 to 2 minutes. Expel the garlic and dispose of. Increment the warmth to high and include the couscous. Cook, blending continually, for 6 minutes. Keep on cooking the couscous, blending like clockwork, until toasted, around 25 minutes. Move the couscous to a huge serving bowl and cool for 5 minutes. Include the ricotta salata, cucumber, sun-dried tomatoes, Parmesan, and basil.

3.For the dressing: In a little bowl, whisk together the oil, lemon juice, lemon pizzazz, salt, and pepper until smooth.

4.Pour the dressing over the serving of mixed greens and hurl until the couscous is covered.

Tomato Fennel Salad

- Complete: 10 min
- Prep: 10 min
- Yield: 6 to 8 servings

Fixings

1/2 pounds treasure tomatoes
1 little fennel bulb
2 tablespoons great olive oil
2 tablespoons new lemon juice
1 tablespoon juice vinegar
1 teaspoon genuine salt
  1/2 teaspoon crisply ground dark pepper

Bearings

1.Center the tomatoes and cut into wedges. Expel the highest point of the fennel (spare a few fronds for embellishment) and cut the bulb all around meagerly transversely with a blade or on a mandoline.

2.Hurl the tomatoes and fennel in a bowl with the olive oil, lemon juice, vinegar, salt, and pepper. Enhancement with 2 tablespoons cleaved fennel fronds, season to taste, and serve.

Chocolate Orange Mousse

- All out: 20 hr 35 min
- Prep: 35 min
- Idle: 20 hr
- Yield: 6 to 8 servings

Fixings

6 ounces great semisweet chocolate, cleaved
2 ounces great clashing chocolate, cleaved

1/4 cup orange alcohol (prescribed: Grand Marnier)
1/4 cup water
1 teaspoon unadulterated vanilla concentrate
1 teaspoon ground orange pizzazz
12 tablespoons (1/2 sticks) unsalted margarine, at room temperature
8 extra-enormous eggs, at room temperature, isolated
1/2 cup in addition to 2 tablespoons sugar
Squeeze fit salt
1/2 cup cold overwhelming cream
Whipped Cream, formula pursues, for improvement
   Mandarin oranges, depleted, for improvement

Whipped Cream:

2 cups (1 16 ounces) cold substantial cream
2 tablespoons sugar
   Dash unadulterated vanilla concentrate

Bearings

1.Consolidate the 2 chocolates, orange alcohol, 1/4 cup water, and the vanilla in a warmth proof bowl. Set it over a dish of stewing water just until the chocolate liquefies. Cool totally to room temperature. Race in the orange get-up-and-go and spread until consolidated.

2.Spot the egg yolks and 1/2 cup of the sugar in the bowl of an electric blender fitted with the oar connection. Beat on rapid for 4 minutes, or until extremely thick and light yellow. With the blender on low speed, include the chocolate blend. Move to an enormous bowl.

3.Spot 1 cup of egg whites (spare or dispose of the rest), the salt, and 1 tablespoon of the sugar in the bowl of an electric blender fitted with the whisk connection. Beat on fast until firm however not dry. Whisk 1/4 of the egg whites into the chocolate blend; at that point overlay the rest in cautiously with an elastic spatula.

4.Without cleaning the bowl or whisk, whip the overwhelming cream and the rest of the tablespoon of sugar until firm. Overlap the whipped cream into the chocolate blend. Empty the mousse into individual dishes or a 8-cup serving bowl. Chill and adorn with whipped cream and oranges. Present with extra whipped cream as an afterthought.

Whipped Cream:

1.Whip the cream in the bowl of an electric blender fitted with the whisk connection. When it begins to thicken, include the sugar and vanilla and keep on whipping until the cream shapes hardened pinnacles. Don't overbeat, or you'll wind up with margarine!

Barbecued Skirt Steak with Smoky Herb Sauce

- All out: 45 min (incorporates resting time)
- Dynamic: 35 min
- Yield: 4 servings

Fixings

Steak:

One 1-pound skirt steak or flank steak
1 teaspoon fit salt
1 tablespoon olive oil
   1/2 lemon

Herb Sauce:

1 shallot, minced
1/3 cup pressed crisp basil leaves, hacked
1/3 cup pressed crisp mint leaves, hacked
   1/3 cup pressed crisp Italian parsley leaves, hacked

1/2 cup extra-virgin olive oil
3/4 teaspoon fit salt
1 teaspoon ground lemon pizzazz

1 tablespoon lemon juice

1/4 cup cut almonds, toasted and hacked

3/4 teaspoon smoked paprika

Bearings

1.For the steak: Preheat a flame broil or barbecue container to medium high.

2.Sprinkle the skirt steak with the salt and shower with the olive oil. Spot on the flame broil and cook to the ideal doneness, 4 to 6 minutes for each side, contingent upon the thickness. (The outside of the steak ought to have a brilliant darker scorch.) Remove to a platter and crush the lemon half over the steak. Let rest for 10 minutes.

3.For the herb sauce: Meanwhile, put the shallot, basil, mint, parsley, olive oil, salt, lemon pizzazz, lemon juice, almonds and paprika in a medium bowl. Combine until consolidated.

4.Cut the steak on the inclination into 1/2-inch-thick cuts, contrary to what would be expected. Present with the herb sauce.

Chilaquiles Rojos (Traditional Mexican Breakfast Dish)

- All out: 1 hr 5 min
- Dynamic: 1 hr 5 min
- Yield: 4 servings

Fixings

10 ready Roma tomatoes, quartered
8 serrano chiles, left entire, stems evacuated
5 cloves garlic, stripped
1 white onion, stripped and quartered
4 tablespoons oil
    Salt
Chicken base, for flavoring
6 ounces tomato puree
8 ounces cooked and destroyed chicken
3 ounces slashed new cilantro, in addition to cilantro sprigs for serving
6 ounces tortilla chips, strips or squares are ideal
6 ounces harsh cream
1 onion, cut into rings
12 ounces disintegrated queso fresco cheddar or panela cheddar Arranged guacamole, for serving
Arranged refried dark beans, for serving
    Arranged pico de gallo salsa, for serving

Headings

1.Barbecue the tomatoes, chiles, garlic and onions until they have a somewhat darkened skin. Try not to consume!

2.Heat 6 cups water to the point of boiling with the darkened veggies until they are cooked through and delicate inside.

3.Pour the veggies with the high temp water and a little included virus water into a nourishment processor and procedure. Try not to mix excessively, you need the blend to be stout.

4.In a huge pot, heat up the oil until smoking. At that point (cautiously!) include a limited quantity of the sauce blend and let it consume with extreme heat for 1 moment (this is for a pleasant smoky flavor). At that point gradually include the remainder of the blend and season with salt and some chicken base.

5.Include the tomato puree for shading, and blend well. Include the destroyed chicken and cook until it is warmed through. Include the cilantro. Include the chips and serve quickly on 4 plates. Top each plate with some sharp cream, cut onions, queso fresco and a sprig of cilantro.

6.Present with guacamole, refried dark beans and pico de gallo as an afterthought.

Cook's Note

The Serrano chiles make this dish extremely fiery! Decrease the measure of chiles for less flavor. Make this morning meal somewhat heartier by serving it with fricasseed or fried eggs on top.

Peach, Corn and Burrata Bruschetta

- All out: 1 hr (incorporates marinating time)
- Dynamic: 30 min
- Yield: 8 servings

Fixings

2 ears corn, bits cut off
2 little peaches, cut into meager wedges
1 Fresno or serrano chile, meagerly cut
1/3 cup slashed new basil
2 teaspoons white balsamic vinegar
1 tablespoon extra-virgin olive oil, in addition to additional for sprinkling, discretionary 1/2 teaspoon fit salt
Eight 1/2-inch-thick cuts crusty bread
1/4 cup olive oil

8 ounces burrata cheddar, depleted and tapped dry
1/2 teaspoon flaky ocean salt

Headings

1.In a medium bowl, join the corn, peaches, chile, basil, white balsamic, extra-virgin olive oil and legitimate salt. Blend well with a spoon. Let marinate for 30 minutes at room temperature or as long as 2 hours in the icebox.

2.In the mean time, heat a flame broil or barbecue skillet over medium-high heat. Shower the crusty bread cuts with the olive oil and flame broil until brilliant dark colored, around 1 moment for each side.

3.To serve, detach modest quantities of burrata and spot on the toast. Sprinkle with the flaky ocean salt. Spoon a portion of the serving of mixed greens on top. Sprinkle with a touch progressively olive oil whenever wanted.

Endive and Avocado Salad

- Absolute: 15 min

- Prep: 15 min
- Yield: 6 servings

Fixings

1/2 tablespoon Dijon mustard
1/4 cup crisply pressed lemon juice (2 lemons)
1/4 cup great olive oil
3/4 teaspoon legitimate salt
1/2 teaspoon newly ground dark pepper
3 heads endive
   3 ready Haas avocados, stripped and seeded

Bearings

1.Whisk together the mustard, lemon juice, olive oil, salt, and pepper to make a vinaigrette. Expel a 1/2-inch from the stem part of the arrangement, dispose of the center, and cut the rest crosswise over into 1-inch pieces. Cut the avocados into enormous shakers or wedges. Hurl the avocados and endive with the vinaigrette. Season, to taste, and serve at room temperature.

2.Note: Haas avocados are the darker ones from California. The green ones don't have so much season.

Flame broiled Melon and Prosciutto Pasta Salad

- Complete: 35 min
- Dynamic: 35 min
- Yield: 6 to 8 servings

Fixings

Dressing:

1 tablespoon Dijon mustard
1/4 cup champagne vinegar
1/2 cup extra-virgin olive oil
1/2 teaspoon legitimate salt
1/4 cup hacked new basil
2 tablespoons hacked Italian parsley
1 tablespoon hacked new tarragon
1/2 cup newly ground Parmesan
Plate of mixed greens:
2 tablespoons olive oil
4 ounces cut prosciutto, cut into dainty strips
1/2 melon, skin expelled, cut into wedges
1 pound farfalle pasta, cooked and cooled
    1 cup set Castelvetrano olives, split

Bearings

1.For the dressing: In a huge bowl, whisk together the mustard, vinegar, extra-virgin olive oil and salt until emulsified. Include the basil, parsley, tarragon and Parmesan and mix to consolidate.

2.For the plate of mixed greens: Heat a medium skillet over medium warmth. Include the olive oil and prosciutto and cook, mixing frequently with a wooden spoon, until the prosciutto is dark colored and fresh, around 6 minutes. Utilizing an opened spoon, evacuate the prosciutto to a paper towel-lined plate. Let cool.

3.Warmth a barbecue dish over high heat. Spot the melon wedges in the dish and flame broil until pleasant barbecue imprints show up and the melon is somewhat caramelized, around 1 moment for every side. Evacuate to a cutting board and slash into reduced down pieces.

4.Include the barbecued melon, pasta and olives to the bowl with the dressing and hurl well to coat. Sprinkle with the firm prosciutto.

Cook's Note

The plate of mixed greens can be refrigerated for multi day before serving. Simply leave off the prosciutto until a minute ago.

Barbecued Artichokes with Parsley and Garlic

- All out: 47 min
- Prep: 25 min
- Cook: 22 min
- Yield: 6 servings

Fixings

6 new artichokes
2 lemons split, in addition to 1/3 cup naturally pressed lemon juice
3 tablespoons newly slashed level leaf parsley
1 teaspoon minced garlic
Salt and newly ground dark pepper
1/2 cup extra-virgin olive oil

Bearings

1.Heat a huge pot of salted water to the point of boiling. Preheat barbecue to medium-high warm.

2.Trim the come from every artichoke to 1-inch long, at that point curve back and snap off dim external leaves. Cut top inch of artichokes with serrated blade. Utilizing a vegetable peeler, strip dull green zones from stem and base of artichoke. Quarter every artichoke.

167

Utilizing a little, sharp blade, cut out the stifle and expel the purple, thorny tipped leaves from the focal point of each wedge.

3.Spot completed artichokes in an enormous bowl of virus water and crush 2 lemons into the water and blend. Proceed with outstanding artichokes.

4.When completed, channel the artichokes and spot into bubbling water and cook until fresh delicate, around 12 minutes.

5.Channel the cooked artichokes and spot onto preheated flame broil. Cook until delicate and gently scorched in spots, turning once in a while, around 10 minutes.

6.In the mean time, in a medium measured bowl, include remaining lemon juice (1/3 cup) parsley, garlic and salt and pepper, to taste. Bit by bit shower in olive oil.

7.Hurl or sprinkle the barbecue artichokes with the garlic/parsley blend and serve.

Cherry Balsamic Chicken

- All out: 3 hr 25 min (incorporates marinating and sitting occasions)

- Dynamic: 25 min
- Yield: 4 servings

Fixings

1 cup jolted sweet fruits
1/4 cup balsamic vinegar
1 tablespoon Dijon mustard
1 teaspoon fennel seed, toasted
1 teaspoon genuine salt
1 clove garlic, crushed and stripped
One 3 1/2-pound chicken, cut into 8 pieces
2 tablespoons olive oil
   1/2 teaspoon fennel dust or ground toasted fennel
   seed

Headings

1.Join the fruits, vinegar, mustard, fennel seed, salt and garlic in a blender. Puree until smooth. Spot the chicken pieces in a resealable plastic pack and pour the marinade over the chicken. Seal the sack and hurl to coat. Marinate in the cooler for 2 hours.

2.Expel the chicken from the cooler 30 minutes before flame broiling. Preheat a flame broil to 450 degrees F or medium-high heat with backhanded warmth on one side.

3.Expel the chicken pieces from the marinade and spot on a heating sheet; save the marinade. Shower with the olive oil. Spot the chicken on the barbecue over direct warmth and cook undisturbed for 4 minutes. Flip the chicken, move to backhanded warmth and season with the marinade. Spread the flame broil and meal until the chicken is cooked through, around 30 minutes. Evacuate to a platter and sprinkle with the fennel dust.

Spanish Spice Rubbed Chicken Breasts with Parsley-Mint Sauce

- Absolute: 45 min
- Prep: 30 min
- Dormant: 5 min
- Cook: 10 min
- Yield: 4 servings

Fixings

Flavor Rubbed Chicken:
1 tablespoon Spanish paprika
1 tablespoon smoked paprika

2 teaspoons cumin seeds, ground

2 teaspoons mustard seeds, ground

2 teaspoons fennel seeds, ground

1 teaspoon coarsely ground dark pepper

2 teaspoons genuine salt

4 (8-ounce) boneless chicken bosoms

Olive oil

Parsley-Mint Sauce, formula pursues

Parsley-Mint Sauce:

1/2 cups firmly stuffed new mint leaves

3/4 cup firmly stuffed new level leaf parsley

6 cloves garlic, cleaved

2 serrano chiles, flame broiled, stripped, hacked

2 tablespoons necta

2 tablespoons Dijon mustard

1 cup olive oil

Water

Salt and crisply ground dark pepper

Bearings

1.Preheat your flame broil to high.

2.Whisk together the paprika, cumin, mustard, fennel, pepper and salt in a little bowl.

3.Brush the chicken with a couple of teaspoons of oil on the two sides. Rub the bosoms on the skin side with a portion of the rub and spot on the flame broil, rub side down. Flame broil until brilliant darker and marginally scorched, 4 to 5 minutes. Turn the bosoms over and keep cooking until simply cooked through, 4 to 5 minutes. Move the chicken to a platter and promptly shower with a portion of the Parsley-Mint Sauce. Let rest 5 minutes. Present with extra sauce as an afterthought.

Parsley-Mint Sauce:

1.Spot the mint, parsley, garlic and serranos in a sustenance processor and procedure until coarsely cleaved. Include the nectar and mustard and procedure until joined. With the engine running, gradually include the olive oil until emulsified.

2.Move the blend to a bowl and race in a couple of tablespoons of virus water to thin to a sauce-like consistency. Season with salt and pepper to taste.

Mediterranean Halibut Sandwiches

- All out: 50 min
- Prep: 15 min
- Idle: 20 min
- Cook: 15 min

- Yield: 4 sandwiches

Fixings

Fish:

Vegetable oil cooking shower
1 (12-ounce) or 2 (6-ounce) focus cut halibut filets,
cleaned 1/2 teaspoon fit salt
1/4 teaspoon naturally ground dark pepper
Extra-virgin olive oil, for sprinkling

Bread:

1 portion crusty bread, closes cut, divided the long
way
2 tablespoons extra-virgin olive oil
1 clove garlic, stripped and divided

Filling:

1/3 cup mayonnaise
1/4 cup slashed sun-dried tomatoes
1/4 cup slashed new basil leaves
2 tablespoons slashed new parsley leaves
1 tablespoon escapades, depleted
Pizzazz of 1 huge lemon
1/2 teaspoon fit salt
1/4 teaspoon naturally ground dark pepper

2 cups arugula

Headings

1.For the fish: Place a broiler rack in the focal point of the stove. Preheat the stove to 450 degrees F. Splash a little heating sheet or glass preparing dish with vegetable oil cooking shower. Put in a safe spot.

2.Season the halibut on the two sides with the salt and pepper. Spot on the heating sheet and shower with oil. Prepare until the fish is cooked through and the tissue drops effectively with a fork, 10 to 15 minutes. Put aside to cool totally, around 20 minutes.

3.For the bread: Preheat a flame broil dish or a huge nonstick skillet over medium-high heat. Expel a portion of the mixture from the top portion of the bread. Brush the cut-sides of the bread with olive oil. Flame broil the bread until brilliant, 1 to 2 minutes, and rub the cooked surface with the cut side of the garlic.

4.For the filling: In a medium bowl, consolidate the mayonnaise, sun-dried tomatoes, basil, parsley, tricks, lemon pizzazz, salt, and pepper.

5.Utilizing a fork, chip the cooked fish and add to the filling. Blend until fused. Spot the filling on the base portion of the bread. Top with arugula. Include the top portion of the bread and cut into 4 equivalent estimated sandwiches.

Marsh Cabbage

- All out: 25 min
- Prep: 5 min
- Cook: 20 min
- Yield: 8 to 10 side servings

Fixings

3 cuts bacon
2 heads crisply cut marsh cabbage (hearts of palm),
hacked 1/2 cup sugar
1 tablespoon salt
   1/2 tablespoon naturally ground dark pepper

Headings

1.In a medium pan, fry the bacon over medium
warmth. Put in a safe spot, holding drippings. Put bog
cabbage and remaining fixings, including seared bacon
and bacon drippings, in a 6-quart pot. Fill the pot 1/2
full with water and heat to the point of boiling. Keep on
bubbling for 10 to 15 minutes, until the cabbage is

delicate. Modify salt and pepper, to taste. Serve hot as a side dish.

Cook's Note

In the case of warming remains, you should bring to a full bubble once more.

Tortilla Espanola (Spanish Omelet)

- Absolute: 45 min
- Prep: 15 min
- Cook: 30 min
- Yield: 4 servings

Fixings

1/2 cup vegetable oil
4 potatoes, daintily cut
1 white onion, hacked
4 eggs, mixed in a huge bowl
1/4 teaspoon salt
2 to 3 tablespoons extra-virgin olive oil

Bearings

1.In a huge skillet over medium-high heat, include the vegetable oil until the dish is filled midway. When the oil is hot, include the potato cuts and onion, ensuring they are well-shrouded by the oil; include more oil if important. Cook for 20 minutes until the potatoes and onions are delicate. Channel the oil and join the potato blend with the eggs. Include the salt and blend well.

2.In a 10-inch by 2 1/2 inch nonstick skillet, include the olive oil and warmth over medium-high heat. Pour in the potato, egg, and onion blend. Lower the warmth to medium-low and cook for 4 to 5 minutes, until the base of the omelet is light darker. Utilizing a level fired plate, spread the griddle and flip the omelet over onto the plate. Quickly slip the uncooked side again into the dish. Cook for another 4 to 5 minutes, until the opposite side is a light dark colored.

3.Expel the omelet from the container to a plate and cut into 4 wedges.

Bar-b-que Vegetable Medley

- All out: 55 min
- Prep: 20 min
- Idle: 10 min
- Cook: 25 min
- Yield: 4 to 6 servings

Fixings

1/4 cup olive oil
1 green ringer pepper, cut
1 red ringer pepper, cut
1 yellow ringer pepper, cut
10 little tomatoes, cut
1 red onion, cut
1 crookneck squash, cut
1 zucchini, cut
1/2 cup crisp basil leaves, cleaved
    Salt
    Dark pepper

Headings

1.Pour the oil in an enormous bowl and include the peppers, tomatoes, onion, squash, zucchini, and basil in a bowl and hurl to consolidate. Season with salt and pepper, to taste. Give vegetables a chance to represent

10 minutes before putting them into a BBQ wok bushel.

2.Warmth the flame broil to medium. Spot vegetables (in the wok container) on the flame broil and cook, blending sporadically. Expel the vegetables from the flame broil and serve right away.

The Ultimate Grilled Shrimp

- All out: 25 min
- Prep: 15 min
- Cook: 10 min
- Yield: 4 servings

Fixings

Oil
1 cup (2 sticks) unsalted margarine, relaxed
1 bundle crisp basil leaves
2 lemons, partitioned
Genuine salt and naturally ground dark pepper
16 enormous head-on kind sized shrimp in the shell, shells split down the back

Headings

1.Put an enormous barbecue container on 2 burners over medium-high heat or preheat an open air gas or charcoal flame broil and get it hot. In case you're utilizing an open air flame broil, take a couple of paper towels and overlap them more than a few times to make a thick square. Smudge a limited quantity of oil on the paper towel, at that point cautiously and rapidly wipe the hot meshes of the flame broil to make a nonstick barbecuing surface.

2.In the interim, include the margarine into a sustenance processor with the basil leaves (save a couple for enhancement), the juice of 1 of the lemons, and salt and pepper. Puree. Stuff about portion of the margarine under the shells of the shrimp (around 1/2 tablespoon for every shrimp). Lay the shrimp on the hot flame broil and cook for 3 minutes on each side, brushing with the rest of the basil margarine a couple of times as they cook.

3.To serve, put the shrimp on plates and speck with the rest of the basil spread. Press the rest of the lemon over the shrimp and trimming the plates with basil leaves.

Thyme Pasta Frittata

- Complete: 19 min
- Prep: 5 min
- Cook: 14 min
- Yield: 4 to 6 servings

Fixings

6 eggs
3 tablespoons whipping cream
1 cup ground Parmesan
3 cups cooked and cooled penne pasta
3 tablespoons coarsely hacked crisp thyme leaves
2 tablespoons hacked crisp level leaf parsley
1 lemon, zested
1/2 teaspoon legitimate salt
1/2 teaspoon newly ground dark pepper
    2 tablespoons olive oil

Bearings

1.In a huge bowl, whisk together the eggs and cream. Blend in the cheddar, pasta, 2 tablespoons of the thyme, parsley, lemon get-up-and-go, salt, and pepper.

181

2.In a 10-inch nonstick skillet, heat the oil over medium warmth. Empty the egg blend into the dish and cook for 7 to 8 minutes until the edges start to darker. Expel the dish from the warmth. Utilizing a spatula, slide the frittata onto a supper plate. Cautiously reverse the frittata again into the skillet and keep on cooking until firm, 5 to 6 minutes

3.Enhancement with the rest of the thyme. Cut into wedges and serve warm or at room temperature.

Flame broiled Shrimp

- All out: 15 min
- Prep: 5 min
- Cook: 10 min
- Yield: 4 servings

Fixings

2 enormous cloves of garlic, cleaved

1/2 cup extra-virgin olive oil

16 enormous head-on kind sized shrimp in the shell, shells split down the back Genuine salt and crisply ground dark pepper

Headings

1.Warmth an enormous open air flame broil and wipe down with oiled paper towel to make a nonstick surface. Add slashed garlic to 1/2 cup oil. Season shrimp with salt and pepper and spot on flame broil. Treat with garlic-olive oil and flame broil 3 minutes each side seasoning as you go.

Block Oven-Style Chicken

- All out: 1 hr 20 min (incorporates resting time)
- Dynamic: 25 min
- Yield: 4 servings

Fixings

1/2 teaspoons genuine salt
1/8 teaspoon crisply ground dark pepper

1 teaspoon cleaved new thyme

1 teaspoon ground lemon pizzazz

One 3-pound chicken, spatchcocked or cut into 8 pieces

3 Roma tomatoes, split or quartered

2 fennel bulbs, cut into 8 wedges each

3 tablespoon olive oil

2 tablespoons cleaved new basil

Bearings

1.Preheat the stove to 500 degrees F.

2.In a little bowl, combine the salt, pepper, thyme and lemon get-up-and-go. Sprinkle the chicken on the two sides with everything except 1/2 teaspoon of the blend. Spot the chicken skin-side up in an enormous (5-quart) braiser or cast-iron skillet. Settle the tomato parts and fennel wedges around the chicken; season the vegetables with the staying salt blend. Sprinkle the chicken and vegetables with the olive oil.

3.Spread the container and spot in the stove for 20 minutes. Reveal and come back to the broiler for about an additional 20 minutes, until the chicken is brilliant darker and a moment read thermometer embedded into the thickest piece of the bosom peruses 160 degrees F. Let rest for 15 minutes before cutting.

4.Serve the chicken close by the vegetables, showered with dish squeezes and sprinkled with the basil.

Taco Burgers

- Complete: 15 min
- Dynamic: 15 min
- Yield: 8 servings

Fixings

2 pounds ground meat toss
1 tablespoon legitimate salt
1 tablespoon cumin
2 teaspoons smoked paprika
1 tablespoon olive oil
1 heart of romaine lettuce, finely cut
4 potato burger buns, toasted
1 cup destroyed Cheddar
1 on-the-vine tomato, cut
Cured jalapenos, for garnish, discretionary
Sharp cream, for garnish, discretionary

Bearings

1.Preheat a flame broil or barbecue dish to medium-high warm.

2.In a medium bowl, combine the hurl, salt, cumin and paprika. Gap into 4 even patties and shower with a pinch of olive oil. Barbecue the burgers until profound darker and marginally cooked through, 3 to 4 minutes for every side.

3.Heap a bed of lettuce on the base of every bun. Top with a patty, some cheddar and a cut of tomato. Top with cured jalapenos and acrid cream whenever wanted.

Bacalaitos (Codfish Fritters)

- Complete: 50 min
- Prep: 10 min
- Cook: 40 min
- Yield: 30 squanders

Fixings

1/2 pound salted cod, absorbed medium-term 3 cups of milk
4 1/2 cups water
3 cups milk
1/2 cups flour
1 teaspoon heating powder
1 little onion, 1/2-inch dice
1 little sweet red pepper, 1/2-inch dice
2 cloves garlic, squashed
1/2 bundle cilantro, cleaved
    Oil, for fricasseeing

Headings

1.Channel salted cod. Bubble fish in 3 cups of the water and the milk until delicate, around 20 to 30 minutes. Expel cooked fish from fluid, shred and put aside to cool. Make a player with the flour, preparing powder and remaining water. Include cod, onions, peppers, garlic and cilantro. Profound fry spoonfuls of the hitter in oil warmed to 350 degrees until brilliant.

Li Hing Margarita

- Absolute: 5 min
- Prep: 5 min
- Yield: 1 beverage

Fixings

1/2 ounces tequila (suggested: Coaps Reposado)
1/2-ounce orange-seasoned alcohol (suggested: Cointreau)
1-ounce lime juice
1/2 ounces sweet and sharp blend
1/2-ounce mango puree
    2 teaspoons li hing mui powder

Bearings

1.Fill a blender with ice, include every one of the fixings, aside from the powder, and mix. Edge a glass with li hing mui powder and serve right away.

Toasted Baguette

- Absolute: 20 min

- Prep: 5 min
- Cook: 15 min
- Yield: 20 to 25 toasts
-

Fixings

1 loaf
1/4 cup olive oil
Legitimate salt
   Newly ground dark pepper

Bearings

1.Preheat the stove to 400 degrees F.

2.Cut the loaf corner to corner into 1/4-inch cuts. You ought to have 20 to 25 cuts. Spot the cuts in 1 layer on a heating sheet. Brush each cut with olive oil and sprinkle with salt and pepper.

3.Heat the toasts for 15 to 20 minutes or until they are fresh and seared. Serve at room temperature.

Korean-style BBQ Short Ribs

- All out: 2 hr 50 min

- Prep: 20 min
- Idle: 2 hr
- Cook: 30 min
- Yield: 4 servings

Fixings

4 enormous short ribs
2 scallions, cleaved
3 garlic cloves, minced
1/2 cup soy sauce
1/4 cup sesame oil
1 teaspoon sesame seeds
2 tablespoons sugar
1/4 teaspoon dark pepper
1 tablespoon purpose (prescribed: Han Soju)
   Cucumber Kimchi, formula pursues, discretionary

Cucumber Kimchi:
5 little pickling cucumbers
2 tablespoons salt
2 cups water
1 pound Chinese turnips, some julienned and some cut
into circles 1/4 cup julienned carrot
2 cloves garlic, minced
2 scallions, julienned
3 hot red peppers, seeded and minced

1 teaspoon minced crisp ginger

1 teaspoon sugar

1 teaspoon salt

3/4 teaspoon cayenne pepper

   1 cup chicken stock

Headings

1.Score ribs each 1/2-inch along the length and width of the bone, trying not to cut excessively profound so the meat will remain connected deep down.

2.Consolidate the rest of the fixings in a bowl to make the marinade. Pour the marinade over the ribs and push the sauce into the cuts so it gets right down deep down. Turn the ribs over face down in the marinade and spread for at least 2 hours or refrigerate medium-term for a more grounded flavor.

3.Expel ribs from the marinade and grill over a charcoal barbecue. Serve ribs with Cucumber Kimchi, steamed rice, and green Korean peppers. Appreciate!

Cucumber Kimchi:

1.Make 3 profound cuts of equivalent size along the length of the cucumbers. Make a point not to slice right to the part of the bargain to keep the cucumbers entirety.

2.Break up the 2 tablespoons of salt in the water. Splash the cucumbers for 2 hours to mellow so they won't split when they get stuffed.

3.For the stuffing, consolidate the rest of the fixings with the exception of the chicken stock and blend well.

4.Press however much water as could reasonably be expected out of the cucumbers. Stuff the turnip blend firmly into the cuts. Spot the cucumbers in a container with the rest of the stuffing and let sit for 3hours. Pour the chicken stock over the cucumbers and let remain at room temperature for 24 hours. Refrigerate and present with Korean short ribs.